The Menopausal Transition

Key Issues in Mental Health

Vol. 175

Series Editors

A. Riecher-Rössler Basel
M. Steiner Hamilton

The Menopausal Transition

Interface between Gynecology and Psychiatry

Volume Editors

Claudio N. Soares Hamilton, Ont.
Michelle Warren New York, N.Y.

9 figures, 4 in color, and 5 tables, 2009

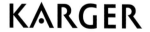
Basel · Freiburg · Paris · London · New York · Bangalore ·
Bangkok · Shanghai · Singapore · Tokyo · Sydney

Key Issues in Mental Health

Formerly published as 'Bibliotheca Psychiatrica' (founded 1917)

Claudio N. Soares
Academic Head
Mood Disorders Division
Director, WHCC
301 James St South, FB 638
L8P 3B6 Hamilton, Ont. (Canada)

Michelle Warren
Dept. of Ob/Gyn, PH 16-20
Columbia University
622 West 168th Street
10032 New York N.Y. (USA)

Library of Congress Cataloging-in-Publication Data

The menopausal transition : interface between gynecology and psychiatry / volume editors, Claudio Soares, Michelle Warren.
    p. ; cm.– (Key issues in mental health, ISSN 1662-4874 ; v. 175)
    Includes bibliographical references and indexes.
    ISBN 978-3-8055-9101-0 (hard cover : alk. paper)
    1. Menopause–Psychological aspects. 2. Perimenopause–Psychological aspects. 3. Middle-aged women–Mental health. I. Soares, Claudio N. II. Warren, Michelle P. III. Series: Key issues in mental health ; v. 175.
    [DNLM: 1. Menopause–psychology. 2. Aging. 3. Depressive Disorder–psychology. W1 B1429 v.175 2009 / WP 580 M5475 2009]
    RG186.M428 2009
    618.1'75–dc22
                            2009003860

Bibliographic Indices. This publication is listed in bibliographic services, including Current Contents®

© Copyright 2009 by S. Karger AG, P.O. Box, CH–4009 Basel (Switzerland)
www.karger.com
Printed in Switzerland on acid-free and non-aging paper (ISO 9706) by Reinhardt Druck, Basel
ISSN 1662–4874
ISBN 978–3–8055–9101–0
e-ISBN 978–3–8055–9102–7

Contents

Foreword

The interplay between the hormone milieu, physiologic changes and psychological symptoms across the female life cycle has long intrigued scientists and physicians. After all, women appear to be particularly vulnerable to the development of psychiatric conditions during certain periods in life that are marked not only by intense – sometimes chaotic – hormone variations and psychosocial stressors but also accompanied by changes in social, family and professional roles in life. For several decades, health professionals and researchers in women's health and psychiatry have attempted to explore the epidemiology, clinical characteristics and underlying mechanisms that contribute to various medical and psychiatric conditions during these 'windows of vulnerability' in a woman's life. Albeit important, isolated efforts have produced limited understanding of the complex nature of these phenomena. Fortunately, more and more investigators have become increasingly aware of the importance of knowledge exchange and integrated research when dealing with female-specific somatic and psychological conditions.

The menopausal transition poses a particular challenge to professionals in psychiatry and gynecology and such a challenge demands an integrated effort. Thus, we conceptualized this book to close the gap in clinical and research knowledge while examining the menopausal transition from an integrated angle of psychologists, psychiatrists, gynecologists, endocrinologists, epidemiologists, etc. The book begins with an overview of 'what to expect' from the menopause transition and its interface with the aging process. Next, relevant but still understudied aspects of the menopausal transition – sexuality, sociocultural changes, impact of life stressors, and emergence of depression are explored. This is followed by reviews of the physiology of thermoregulation and the occurrence of hot flashes; a better understanding of vasomotor complaints is essential given the prevalence and significant burden associated with these symptoms and their putative links to mood changes and sleep disruption. The management of mood and anxiety during the menopausal transition is tackled by offering an update on hormonal and nonhormonal treatment strategies, followed by a discussion on the emergence of psychotic symptoms associated with changes in sex hormones during the peri- and postmenopausal years. Finally, an excellent review on the pros and cons of menopausal hormone therapies in the post-WHI era is offered.

We hope that the information presented here will be clinically useful to all professionals involved in the management of symptomatic, menopausal women and foster further research collaborations in this field.

Claudio N. Soares
Michelle Warren
Volume Editors

Soares CN, Warren M (eds): The Menopausal Transition. Interface between Gynecology and Psychiatry.
Key Issues in Mental Health. Basel, Karger, 2009, vol 175, pp 1–17

Normal Aging and the Menopausal Transition: What to Expect

Nanette Santoro · Genevieve Neal-Perry

Division of Reproductive, Endocrinology, Albert Einstein College of Medicine, Bronx, N.Y., USA

Abstract

The menopausal transition occurs at a wide variety of ages in normal women. Menopause that occurs very early in life (prior to age 40) or very late in life (over age 54) appears to be associated with less than optimal health outcomes. Against the backdrop of reproductive aging, somatic aging is progressing, for the most part in a linear fashion. However, menopause interacts with somatic aging in several ways. The first of these is by making a temporary impact on health. This can be seen by the increases in mood disturbances and new-onset depression associated with the transition to menopause. Another way in which the transition may affect age-related risk of disease is by causing an acceleration of what has, until now, been a more or less linear or stable process. Recent data suggest that adverse metabolic changes concurrent with menopause produce a particularly ominous combination of risks for subsequent cardiovascular disease, and the appearance of the metabolic syndrome at mid-life may accelerate the incidence curve for heart disease. On the other hand, adverse health problems such as migraine headache improve dramatically after traversal of the menopause. Current longitudinal studies are providing important insights into these relationships.

Copyright © 2009 S. Karger AG, Basel

Menopause both transects and interacts with the aging process. Generalized or 'somatic' aging influences the tempo of reproductive aging and the opposite may also be true: that reproductive aging has an impact on the somatic aging process. The recent convergences of large-scale, epidemiological studies of the menopausal transition both in US-based [1] and other [2, 3] cohorts of women have helped clarify the nature of these relationships. This chapter will focus on the reproductive milestones of the menopausal transition and the concurrent age-related changes in physical function, nonreproductive hormones and metabolism. Finally, the long-term relationships between reproductive function and longevity will be examined based upon data taken from postmenopausal cohorts.

What Drives the Normal Menopausal Transition?

Follicular depletion drives ovarian senescence in humans and subhuman primates. This situation may differ from that in rodents, who do not undergo critical decreases in follicular reserve. Recent data in the mouse identifying germline stem cells in adult animals [4] has not been reproduced in women. Ovarian reserve is the major predictor of the age at which natural menopause will occur. Toxic exposures to agents that destroy ovarian follicles such as smoking [1], ionizing radiation, medically treated depression [5], low socioeconomic status [6] and possibly galactose consumption [7] have all been shown to reduce the reproductive life span of women. Exogenous, anatomical challenges to the ovary such as repeated infections and surgeries reduce ovarian reserve [8]. Unilateral oophorectomy advances menopause by about 1–2 years [9]. Hysterectomy with complete ovarian conservation has been reported to have a similar effect [10], suggesting that surgical devitalization of pelvic tissues is the cause of earlier menopause in these cases.

The numbers of oocytes contained within primordial follicle structures in the ovary have been assessed by follicle counting in histological sections of human ovaries. The oocyte complement is at its lifetime maximum at midgestation in fetal life, with a maximum of almost 6–8 million primordial follicles present. These follicles undergo a massive wave of atresia such that by birth, 1–2 million remain, and by the onset of puberty and a woman's first menstrual period, only about 500,000 follicles at present in the ovary. At the beginning of the menopausal transition, when a woman first notes a break in menstrual cyclicity, there are about 25,000 follicles left in her ovaries [11]. By her final menses, there are 1,000 or less [12]. Although structurally normal appearing follicles are still present in the ovary after the final menstrual period, they seldom grow and even more rarely ovulate. A woman who is over the age of 45 and has experienced 12 months of amenorrhea is 90% likely never to have another menstrual period again [13]. It should be remembered, however, that women younger than 45 have a much lower likelihood of having permanent amenorrhea. This finding has been taken to indicate that somatic aging plays a role in helping to finalize ovarian aging. In other words, a younger age at follicle depletion mitigates the process of menopause.

Exposures that protect ovarian longevity include long-term use of oral contraceptives, and other treatments or physiological states that prevent the latter stages of follicle maturation and ovulation [14]. The protective mechanism at play in this scenario appears to be reducing gonadotropin stimulation of the ovary and induction of a relatively hypogonadotropic, hypogonadal state.

What Reproductive Changes Accompany the Transition?

Changes in Menstrual Cycles

The menopausal transition (MT) describes the process by which a woman goes from a state of normal cyclicity to an ultimate state of permanent hypergonadotropic hypogonadism and amenorrhea. The bulk of current information about the transition is based upon the study of women who had regular, monthly menstrual periods during their midreproductive lives. Women with oligoamenorrhea and women who have had hysterectomies represent sizeable portions of the population, but little is known about their menopausal experience. Likewise, there are almost no population-based data on women who undergo an unusually early menopause, i.e. prior to age 45.

The Massachusetts Women's Health Study [1, 15] and the Melbourne Women's Health Project [16] both helped define the cycle changes that accompany menopause. These definitions have proven to be relatively robust across studies [17] and have been supported in the Study of Women's Health Across the Nation (SWAN), a multi-center epidemiological study of over 3,000 American women from 5 different ethnic backgrounds (Caucasian, African-American, Chinese-American, Japanese-American and Hispanic).

The onset of the transition is a perceived change in menstrual cycle length of >7 days, or a skipped cycle. These types of cycle changes identify the early menopause transition, which is the more variable portion of the process. The early transition can be unnoticed or can last for years. It is not accompanied by significant losses of circulating estrogen and, in several studies, estrogen levels have been noted to be normal or even elevated relative to midreproductive aged, cycling women. The late menopausal transition is best defined by > or = 60 days of amenorrhea and heralds in the period of life where estrogen levels become lower. Symptoms associated with menopause, such as hot flashes or vaginal dryness, typically appear or worsen during the late transition. Loss of bone density is first noted at this stage of the transition and not before [18]. Women who experience prolonged amenorrhea are more likely to complete their menopausal transition sooner, especially if they have a very elevated follicle-stimulating hormone (FSH) level [17].

Reproductive Hormonal Changes

Several epidemiological studies have assessed the yearly [19–21] or biannual [22] changes in circulating reproductive hormones drawn from the follicular phase or throughout the menstrual cycle [23]. These studies indicate that estradiol declines and FSH rises with increasing menstrual irregularity. The fact that FSH rises well before there is a measurable decline in estradiol, and while there is even evidence that estradiol is increased [24, 25], indicates that loss of negative feedback from reduced estradiol cannot be the cause of this change in FSH. There is a strong temporal association between the loss of inhibin [19], a granulosa cell produced peptide that restrains FSH secretion, and the onset of the menopause transition. Inhibin is a dimeric hormone molecule that consists of a common alpha subunit and one of two beta subunits. The hormones are members of the transforming growth factor-β (TGF-β) superfamily, with which they share considerable sequence homology. Inhibin B is a product of small, early antral follicles and is secreted primarily during the early to mid-follicular phase of the cycle. Inhibin A is a product of the dominant follicle, corpus luteum and placenta [26]. Both hormones exert negative feedback on the pituitary and decrease FSH secretion. The inhibins are endocrine hormones, as opposed to the beta homodimers of this peptide family, the activins, which serve as paracrine stimulatory factors and act directly within the pituitary gland. The relative reduction in inhibin feedback on FSH secretion that accompanies reproductive aging is a critical determinant of the changes in the human menstrual cycle that occur through the menopausal transition. The current explanation for the monotropic rise in FSH that is observed throughout the early menopause transition is that the reduced overall numbers of follicles causes a smaller growing pool to be available each month. Since the pool of growing follicles produces inhibin B, this reduction in inhibin B output causes FSH to rise and stimulate the available follicles to grow. In the early menopausal transition, the rise in FSH is sufficient to result in follicle growth. There is evidence that folliculogenesis is accelerated [27], however, and that follicle growth dynamics are altered. For example, studies examining follicle growth directly and comparing findings in perimenopausal women to mid-reproductive aged women have observed that follicles begin to grow earlier, but grow at a slower pace and ovulate at a smaller size [28].

There is a strong and consistent association between the monotropic FSH rise that is the hallmark of the perimenopause and decreased inhibin B concentrations, thought to reflect the diminished number of competent primordial follicles available for recruitment in older reproductive-age women [19, 29–33]. This decrease in the follicular pool chronologically precedes, and probably causes, the classically observed increase in circulating FSH [19, 34, 35]. This makes sense in context of the entire reproductive life span. In large cross-sectional studies, women demonstrate incremental increases in circulating FSH with age, when grouped into decades [36]. The ovarian follicle pool is concomitantly declining throughout life [11, 37, 38]. The primordial follicles generate the available cohort for recruitment and growth in any given cycle. As the overall pool of primordial follicles shrinks over time, there is evidence from numerous ultrasound studies of the ovary that the recruitable pool of small antral follicles available to grow in any given month similarly shrinks [39–41]. This decline is gradual and grows progressively worse, with a possible acceleration of follicle loss during the transition [12]. In the face of a reduced number of available follicles, the monotropic rise in FSH can be viewed as a compensatory process to permit monthly ovulation to continue in the face of reduced follicle numbers. This pattern can continue as FSH progressively rises, i.e. the ovary is in a state of 'compensated failure'. Ultimately, cycles become anovulatory by the late menopausal transition [19, 42]. It appears that the dominant follicles that are selected in this high FSH environment are competent in terms of their steroid and inhibin A secretions [43], but are smaller [28] with fewer granulosa cells per follicle [44]. Luteal function is relatively preserved until the menopausal process becomes advanced. A loss of luteal inhibin A and failure of progesterone production occur relatively later in the transition [19, 29].

There is good evidence that luteal function declines across the transition. This was first shown by Metcalf et al. [45] in a sample of New Zealand women. Others have reported reduced luteal Pdg [24] and luteal inhibin A [30, 31] in older reproductive-age women, using daily urinary and serum sampling, respectively. Not all studies have demonstrated reduced luteal progesterone, however [46, 47]. Landgren et al. [46] examined hormones collected three times per week for 4 weeks on an annual basis in a cohort of 13 women who were followed from 4 to 9 years up to their final menstrual period. Although the proportion of anovulatory cycles increased with progress to menopause, an increase in cycles with low luteal progesterone production was not reported. Most recent data from SWAN indicate that a small decrease in luteal progesterone occurs with progress through the transition, along with an increase in the proportion of anovulatory cycles [48]. As anovulatory cycles increase, they become admixed with intervals of hypoestrogenic cycles that are associated with varying amounts of gonadotropin output [49].

This model of compensated and eventually uncompensated ovarian failure can be schematically presented as 'stages' of reproductive aging. The Stages of Reproductive Aging Workshop (STRAW) classification system provides a point of departure for this type of modeling [50]. STRAW separated reproductive aging into 7 stages: Early, Peak and Late Reproductive Years, Early and Late Menopausal Transition, and Early and Late Postmenopause. As women age, the number of primordial follicles is reduced, and so is the growing pool of follicles. Inhibin B gradually decreases and FSH gradually increases through the Early, Peak, and Late Reproductive stages (stages minus five through minus three). The detectable clinical differences between these stages are primarily related to ease of conception, which is maximal in the Peak years, and begins to decline in the fourth decade of life. Menstrual cycle regularity is preserved. Eventually, FSH is released from restraint by inhibin B and rises, intermittently, Late Reproductive stage (minus three). This biochemical event is clinically silent unless detected during the course of a fertility workup. The Early Menopausal Transition (stage minus two) is marked by increasing irregularity of cycles (more than 7 days' variation) or a skipped menstrual period. Follicular phases shorten by up to 7 days, but ovulation is preserved. Despite the maintenance of relatively normal reproductive hormonal dynamics, the ability of the oocyte to fertilize and grow normally is compromised with age. By the Early Transition, fertility becomes unlikely, even with medical assistance. In the Late Menopausal Transition stage (stage minus one), menstrual cycle length becomes consistently prolonged, the rise in FSH becomes more evident, and the possibility of fertility becomes even more remote. Inhibin A is noticeably decreased, with further decreases in inhibin B and other follicle markers, such as Mullerian inhibiting substance (MIS) to undetectable levels [2].

The final menstrual period (FMP) marks the end of the transition, yet it is a retrospective diagnosis that is only attained after a full 12 months of amenorrhea. Even after this milestone is achieved, a menstrual period is not an uncommon event, and occurs in about 10% of women [13]. For the first year after the FMP, variable excursions of estrogen have been shown to occur [51]. Ovulation and progesterone production, however, is exceedingly unlikely.

The changes in menstrual bleeding that accompany these stages of reproductive aging have recently been characterized. During the Early Transition, cycles can become closer together, such that normal intermenstrual intervals as short as 18 days are not unusual [52]. Since some of these Early Transition cycles have elevated or irregular estrogen production [24, 25], they can result in heavier menstrual periods that last longer. However, once the Late Transition is attained, cycles get farther apart and clinically disruptive bleeding is more likely to be due to anatomic problems such as leiomyomata, adenomyosis or endometrial polyps [53].

What Changes in Symptoms and Physical Function Occur with Traversal of the Menopause?

It is useful for both clinicians and their patients to be aware of which clinical symptoms are likely to occur at which transition stages. Interventions and coping strategies can then be usefully deployed. Women who have an awareness of when their most bothersome symptoms are likely to subside can be empowered in this fashion, and will sometimes choose to endure with simpler, nonpharmacologic and low-risk remedies, if all that is needed is the passage of time. Table 1 provides a summary of common signs and symptoms of the transition and their approximate prevalence and/or severity by transition stage, based upon a variety of population and community based studies.

Are There Biological or Lifestyle Factors that Mitigate the Process?

There are few factors known to affect the oocyte supply. Cigarette smoking is the biggest single epidemiologic factor, accounting for 6–24 months shortening of the reproductive life span [1, 54]. Therefore, smoking cessation, and probably avoidance of second-hand smoke, is a behavioral feature that would be associated with a delay in age at menopause. Toxic exposures such as street drugs, an adverse living environment with social stressors, and exposure to HIV infection all appear to be related to an earlier age at menopause [6, 55]. Racial factors also appear to be related to age at menopause, with Hispanic women having a relatively earlier age at their final menses

Table 1. Common signs and symptoms of the menopause transition and their approximate prevalence by transition stage

Stage	Premenopause	Early	Late	Postmenopause
Hot flashes	+	++	++++	+++
Irritability	+	++++	+++	++
Physical limitations	+	++	+++	++++
Depression	+	++	+++	++
Bone demineralization	–	–	++	+++
Frequent menses	+	+++	+	–
Vaginal dryness/irritation	++	+++	++++	++++
Sexual dysfunction	++	+++	+++-++++	+++-++++
Sleep complaints	++	+++	++++	++++

Data taken from refs. [108–112].

and a greater prevalence of early (age <45) or premature (age <40) menopause [56]. Use of oral contraceptives may lower basal FSH levels and be associated with later age at menopause [57, 58]. Physical activity which reduces midlife weight gain, has not been shown to be a predictor of reproductive longevity, but may well prove to be in current, ongoing longitudinal studies such as SWAN [59].

Genetic studies have elucidated some of the factors responsible for the timing of menopause. In twin studies of mono- and dizygotic twin pairs, the tendency for early and premature menopause are strongly genetically linked, as is age at final menses [60–62]. In one large epidemiological cohort, homozygosity for the Pvu II polymorphism for estrogen receptor (ER) alpha was associated with a FMP 6 months earlier and a more than doubling of the risk of hysterectomy risk compared to women without the Pvu II allele [63].

Are There Useful Biomarkers to Track a Woman's Progress?

It remains difficult to establish prospectively when the final menstrual period will occur. Despite the proliferation of hormonal assays for substances secreted directly by the granulosa cell, and thus believed to be more reflective of the follicular reserve than FSH, which is an indirect measure, no dominant marker has emerged from the clinical literature. Recently, the SWAN study attempted to examine the clinical and biochemical features that were associated with the timing of the FMP [54]. Lifestyle factors, such as cigarette smoking, age and menstrual cycle patterns were for the most part better predictors than were hormones. Interestingly, an elevated as well as a low estradiol were both predictive of a faster time to the FMP. Elevated FSH was also associated with a faster time to FMP. Prior epidemiologic definitions of the menopausal transition stages appear, at present, to be the best clinical markers for predicting the FMP [16, 17].

The concept that there is a superior biochemical test for oocyte numbers that can be used to predict the time to menopause with accuracy has led to a search for a 'menopause blood test'. In most studies to date, FSH has been used to determine follicular reserve. Because of its indirect relationship to the ovary, FSH levels reflect the sum of negative feedback inhibition from both estradiol and inhibin. At present, it appears that inhibin B concentrations decline gradually over time in women, with the shrinking of the available follicle cohort. However, at least in the early menopause transition, estradiol can fluctuate dramatically. It is not surprising that, in SWAN, baseline early follicular phase FSH and both low (<25 pg/ml) and high (>100 pg/ml) estradiol were predictive of a shorter time to the FMP [54]. Another strategy to use FSH levels as predictors of menopause is to dynamically provoke FSH secretion using an antiestrogen challenge with clomiphene citrate. Although FSH levels, both basal and after a clomiphene challenge, are predictive of fertility [64], they are have not been shown to be much superior to menstrual cycle changes as noted above in their association with menopause [2].

It is therefore not surprising that the protein products of granulosa cells have been thought to be more reflective of ovarian supply and might therefore be more direct and superior markers of the menopausal process. Inhibin B has been proposed as a measure of proximity to menopause, but it appears to have similar sensitivity and specificity to FSH as a prognostic marker prior to assisted reproductive technology therapy, and similar limitations to FSH in predicting the FMP. Low inhibin B concentrations (below 45 pg/ml) have been linked to reduced responsiveness to ovulation induction methods and a decreased likelihood of pregnancy [65]; however, this cutoff is not supported by other studies, and there is substantial overlap between pregnant and nonpregnant treatment cycles and baseline inhibin B [66, 67]. Inhibin B levels are also lower during clomiphene citrate challenge tests in women with diminished ovarian reserve [67], and correlate with ovarian response to FSH stimulation [68, 69]; however, the overall positive and negative predictive value of this test does not make it a clinically useful menopause marker.

MIS, or anti-Mullerian hormone (AMH), like inhibin, is another TGF-β family peptide produced by granulosa cells. MIS is produced by early follicles and appears to constitute a more stable measure of follicular reserve, which does not vary with cycle phase [70]. Reductions in MIS have been shown with aging and loss of ovarian reserve, and it is proposed as a superior marker for ovarian reserve [71]. However, as women approach the menopausal transition, the sensitivity of current MIS assays is not sufficient to track the process further [72]. There is also a substantial interaction between MIS, inhibin B and body size, with lower levels of these peptides in women as BMI increases [22, 73]. There may be a need to adjust levels for body size in predictive models.

Table 2. Serum markers of ovarian reserve and their properties

Marker	FSH	Inhibin B	MIS	Inhibin A
Source	pituitary	growing follicles	early growing follicles	corpus luteum and placenta
Timing of measurement	early follicular phase (D2-5)	follicular phase	any time	luteal phase
Earliest change	late reproductive years	early transition	mid reproductive years	late transition
Affected by BMI?	yes	yes	yes	unknown
Detection limit reached	never	late transition	early to late transition	late transition to postmenopause

Taken from refs. [19, 20, 30–32, 113].

Finally, direct observation of the follicle supply is possible using transvaginal ultrasound assessments of antral follicles. Antral follicles that have begun to enter the terminal stages of follicle development can be readily seen on ultrasound because of the fluid-filled follicular space. Counts of antral follicles have been shown to correlate with ovarian responsiveness to exogenous gonadotropin stimulation and have been proposed as another method to determine time to menopause [74].

Because each of these methods has limitations, it is likely that a combination of measurements or serial measurements will be needed to achieve the goal of predicting the FMP. Although biochemical markers other than FSH and estradiol were not used, in the SWAN study it has recently been demonstrated that a combination of menstrual history, hormones, race and lifestyle factors known to influence age at menopause could be combined in a multivariable model to improve the prediction [54]. Widespread application of such methods awaits cost-effectiveness assessments. These data are summarized in table 2.

What Are the Concurrent Changes in Somatic Aging?

Cellular aging reflects an inability to perpetually defend against oxidative stress [75, 76]. There are substantial interindividual differences in resistance to oxidative stress that account for some of the variability in longevity between animals of the same species [77–79]. Environmental factors, such as antioxidant exposure, also influence this process [80], as well the inherent attributes of an individual organism's genetic constitution that makes it resistant to oxidative stress. Outcomes of oxidative stress often result in DNA damage, mutagenesis, cancers, or loss of critical cellular functions [81]. In addition to oxidative stress, chromosomal changes, most importantly increased telomere length, are another property of aging cells [82]. Increased telomeres reduce the efficiency of transcription, thereby reducing the sensitivity of cells to various stimulatory and inhibitory inputs.

At the organ level, aging is associated with vascular compromise. Vascular compromise may contribute to some aspects of reproductive aging. Intramyometrial arteriosclerosis has been observed in women of reproductive age – 37% of women under the age of 30, increasing to 83% in women over the age of 39 who were studied after accidental death [83]. Measures of arterial compromise, such as carotid intimal medial thickness (CIMT) and coronary artery calicification (CAC), a sign of advanced plaque formation, occur increasingly with age but are observed in reproductive-aged women at high risk of subsequent cardiovascular disease [84, 85]. A combination of cellular and vascular deprivation decreases function.

There are hormonal and psychological contributions to senescence that act via the neuroendocrine system. The concept of 'allostatic load' refers to a combination of perceived physiological and pathological stress that can be partially measured and related to risk of disability, disease and even death [86, 87]. In this model, chronic stressors adversely affect overall adaptability and ability to ward off further insult.

Conversely, there are several factors that appear to improve and predict longevity in individuals and populations. In animal studies, caloric restriction has long been demonstrated to increase lifespan, presumably acting by reducing oxidative stress through reduced metabolism [88]. Human studies supporting this notion have not been forthcoming. In genetic studies of centenarians and their offspring, favorable genotypes and phenotypes have been discovered that include preservation of cognitive function [89], absence of cardiovascular diseases or diabetes [90], and high HDL cholesterol [91].

It makes sense to conceptualize aging as having two main contributions. The first are a combination of vulnerability factors – some of which are inescapable, such as progressive oxidative damage, others which are partially modifiable, such as toxic exposures leading to vascular compromise, and others which are genetic, such as predisposition to type 2 diabetes. In dynamic balance with these vulnerabilities are survival factors, including resistance to oxidative stress, favorable genetics (involving cognitive function and cholesterol metabolism), neuroendocrine adaptability, and environmental protection against certain types of stress.

How Does Menopause Interact with Aging?

To consider the interactions between menopause and aging it is helpful to view the loss of oocyte/follicle reserve over time as a process apart from somatic aging. In 'experiments of nature' in which oocyte loss occurs at extremely young ages, there appears to be evidence that oocyte function is somewhat improved. For example, women with premature ovarian failure, who experience oocyte loss and prolonged hypergonadotropic amenorrhea prior to age 40, have frequent evidence of intermittent estrogen production and can conceive, albeit rarely [92]. In contrast, women over the age of 45 years, within the 95% CI for a 'normal' age at menopause, almost never conceive after they have prolonged hypergonadotropic amenorrhea and have a much lower likelihood of ever having another menstrual period [13].

Aging directly affects oocyte and follicle function. As age increases, oocytes, subjected to more cumulative oxidative stress, are more prone to failures of function. Disordered meiotic spindle assembly has been observed in normal women in their 40s compared to younger women in their 20s and 30s [93]. Increased chromosomal errors, such as nondisjunction, occur more frequently. Oocyte telomere length decreases with aging, and is a powerful predictor of reduced ovarian reserve and gametogenic errors [94]. At the CNS level, there is evidence from studies in women [95] that, similar to rodent models, central sex steroid feedback is reduced at the time of the menopausal transition [96], and there is also evidence for disorganization of pulsatile patterns of LH and FSH released from the pituitary [97].

Age-related changes in body composition influence reproductive processes. The increasing insulin resistance and adipose accumulation that accompanies aging may have several adverse reproductive effects. The central body fat patterning that occurs in relation to aging accelerates atherosclerosis [98]. Concomitant, age-related reductions in growth hormone and IGF-1 and in adrenal androgen production – the so-called 'somatopause' and 'adrenopause' [99, 100] – may adversely affect health.

The adrenal changes with aging may impact on generalized functional reserve. The human circadian cortisol pattern includes an early morning rise, followed by a late afternoon nadir. With aging, the afternoon nadir becomes less pronounced, leading to a relative hypercortisolemia [101]. This relative hypercortisolemia has been linked to sleep disturbances in the elderly [102], and has been related to the central body fat accumulation, and increases in blood pressure that accompany aging. Increased cortisol is a powerful predictor of loss of functional reserve – so-called 'allostatic load' – and mortality in the elderly [86].

In some women hypertension, insulin resistance and central fat accumulation have been linked with a fulminant onset of 'syndrome X' phenotype [103], also dubbed 'syndrome W' by Mogul et al. [104]. In this working model, changes in reproductive hormones associated with the menopause transition trigger the development of the metabolic syndrome phenotype over a short period of time. There is support for this notion from the Study of Women's Health Across the Nation, a multi-ethnic study of over 3,000 middle-aged women who are traversing the menopause. In SWAN, traditional risk factors for the metabolic syndrome predicted its prevalence at baseline. However, incident metabolic syndrome developing over the transition was most strongly predicted by the relative androgen excess, i.e. the molar ratio of testosterone to estradiol.

Epidemiological studies also suggest linkage between the processes of reproductive and somatic aging. Premature menopause has been associated with increased risk of cardiovascular disease and mortality in some studies [105]. These data have led to the causal inference that early menopause is responsible for the premature cardiovascular disease, due to estrogen withdrawal early in life and acceleration of atherosclerosis. An alternative explanation is also possible, however. In a large, population-based sample of women, in those with premature menopause, the cardiovascular disease often preceded the diagnosis of menopause [56]. It is possible that the underlying processes that led to the premature cardiovascular disease had a negative impact on ovarian reserve.

Conclusions

The convergence of a series of longitudinal studies over the past two decades has permitted a picture of the menopausal process to emerge. Consistencies across worldwide cohort studies describe a process in which the initial appearance of menstrual irregularity progresses to lengthening of the inter-menstrual interval, accompanied by symptoms of hypoestrogenemia. Hormonal patterns associated with these menstrual cycle changes are being described, with the hope of arriving at serum markers that will predict the progression to the final menstrual period. The majority of women experience transient symptoms associated with the menopause, but endure the process without significant impairment. However, the most recent data indicate that some women are at risk for new onset of a major depression, and others suffer significant bother from their menopausal symptoms of hot flashes and/or vaginal dryness. Sleep can also be negatively affected by the transition. Since symptoms subside for most women, providing support through the process may be all that is necessary. An appreciation of how the aging process intertwines and influences the menopausal transition is important for clinicians, because recognition of adverse phenotypes, e.g. the metabolic syndrome, may allow for early intervention and preventive strategies that will ensure healthy aging.

References

1 McKinlay SM: The normal menopause transition: an overview. Maturitas 1996;23:137–145.
2 Burger HG, Dudley EC, Robertson DM, Dennerstein L: Hormonal changes in the menopause transition. Recent Prog Horm Res 2002;57:257–275.
3 Rossmanith WG, Reichelt C, Scherbaum WA: Neuroendocrinology of aging in humans: attenuated sensitivity to sex steroid feedback in elderly postmenopausal women. Neuroendocrinology 1994; 59:355–362.
4 Johnson J, Canning J, Kaneko T, Pru JK, Tilly JL: Germline stem cells and follicular renewal in the postnatal mammalian ovary. Nature 2004;428:145–150.
5 Harlow BL, Wise LA, Otto MW, Soares CN, Cohen LS: Depression and its influence on reproductive endocrine and menstrual cycle markers associated with perimenopause: the Harvard Study of Moods and Cycles. Arch Gen Psychiatry 2003;60:29–36.

6 Luoto R, Kaprio J, Uutela A: Age at natural meno-pause and sociodemographic status in Finland. Am J Epidemiol 1994;139:64–76.

7 Cooper GS, Hulka BS, Baird DD, et al: Galactose consumption, metabolism, and follicle-stimulating hormone concentrations in women of late repro-ductive age. Fertil Steril 1994;62:1168–1175.

8 Yanushpolsky EH, Best CL, Jackson KV, Clarke RN, Barbieri RL, Hornstein MD: Effects of endometri-omas on oocyte quality, embryo quality, and preg-nancy rates in in vitro fertilization cycles: a prospective, case-controlled study. J Assist Reprod Genet 1998;15:193–197.

9 Cooper GS, Thorp JM Jr: FSH levels in relation to hysterectomy and to unilateral oophorectomy. Obstet Gynecol 1999;94:969–972.

10 Ahn EH, Bai SW, Song CH, et al: Effect of hysterec-tomy on conserved ovarian function. Yonsei Med J 2002;43:53–58.

11 Richardson SJ, Nelson JF: Follicular depletion dur-ing the menopausal transition. Ann N Y Acad Sci 1990;592:13–20; discussion 44–51.

12 Richardson SJ, Senikas V, Nelson JF: Follicular depletion during the menopausal transition: evi-dence for accelerated loss and ultimate exhaustion. J Clin Endocrinol Metab 1987;65:1231–1237.

13 Wallace RB, Sherman BM, Bean JA, Treloar AE, Schlabaugh L: Probability of menopause with increasing duration of amenorrhea in middle-aged women. Am J Obstet Gynecol 1979;135:1021–1024.

14 Cramer DW, Xu H, Harlow BL: Does 'incessant' ovulation increase risk for early menopause? Am J Obstet Gynecol 1995;172:568–573.

15 Brambilla DJ, McKinlay SM, Johannes CB: Defining the perimenopause for application in epidemiologic investigations. Am J Epidemiol 1994;140:1091–1095.

16 Dudley EC, Hopper JL, Taffe J, Guthrie JR, Burger HG, Dennerstein L: Using longitudinal data to define the perimenopause by menstrual cycle char-acteristics. Climacteric 1998;1:18–25.

17 Harlow SD, Crawford S, Dennerstein L, Burger HG, Mitchell ES, Sowers MF: Recommendations from a multi-study evaluation of proposed criteria for stag-ing reproductive aging. Climacteric 2007;10:112–119.

18 Finkelstein JS, Brockwell SE, Mehta V, et al: Bone mineral density changes during the menopause transition in a multi-ethnic cohort of women. J Clin Endocrinol Metab 2007.

19 Burger HG, Dudley EC, Hopper JL, et al: Prospectively measured levels of serum follicle-stimulating hormone, estradiol, and the dimeric inhibins during the menopausal transition in a pop-ulation-based cohort of women. J Clin Endocrinol Metab 1999;84:4025–4030.

20 Randolph JF Jr, Sowers M, Bondarenko IV, Harlow SD, Luborsky JL, Little RJ: Change in estradiol and follicle-stimulating hormone across the early meno-pausal transition: effects of ethnicity and age. J Clin Endocrinol Metab 2004;89:1555–1561.

21 Randolph JF Jr, Sowers M, Gold EB, et al: Reproductive hormones in the early menopausal transition: relationship to ethnicity, body size, and menopausal status. J Clin Endocrinol Metab 2003; 88:1516–1522.

22 Freeman EW, Sammel MD, Gracia CR, et al: Follicular phase hormone levels and menstrual bleeding status in the approach to menopause. Fertil Steril 2005;83:383–392.

23 Ferrell RJ, O'Connor KA, Rodriguez G, et al: Monitoring reproductive aging in a 5-year prospec-tive study: aggregate and individual changes in ste-roid hormones and menstrual cycle lengths with age. Menopause 2005;12:567–577.

24 Santoro N, Brown JR, Adel T, Skurnick JH: Characterization of reproductive hormonal dynam-ics in the perimenopause. J Clin Endocrinol Metab 1996;81:1495–1501.

25 Shideler SE, DeVane GW, Kalra PS, Benirschke K, Lasley BL: Ovarian-pituitary hormone interactions during the perimenopause. Maturitas 1989;11:331–339.

26 Roberts VJ, Barth S, el-Roeiy A, Yen SS: Expression of inhibin/activin subunits and follistatin messen-ger ribonucleic acids and proteins in ovarian folli-cles and the corpus luteum during the human menstrual cycle. J Clin Endocrinol Metab 1993; 77:1402–1410.

27 Klein NA, Battaglia DE, Miller PB, Branigan EF, Giudice LC, Soules MR: Ovarian follicular develop-ment and the follicular fluid hormones and growth factors in normal women of advanced reproductive age. J Clin Endocrinol Metab 1996;81:1946–1951.

28 Santoro N, Isaac B, Neal-Perry G, et al: Impaired folliculogenesis and ovulation in older reproductive aged women. J Clin Endocrinol Metab 2003;88:5502–5509.

29 Klein NA, Illingworth PJ, Groome NP, McNeilly AS, Battaglia DE, Soules MR: Decreased inhibin B secretion is associated with the monotropic FSH rise in older, ovulatory women: a study of serum and follicular fluid levels of dimeric inhibin A and B in spontaneous menstrual cycles. J Clin Endocrinol Metab 1996;81:2742–2745.

30 Reame NE, Wyman TL, Phillips DJ, de Kretser DM, Padmanabhan V: Net increase in stimulatory input resulting from a decrease in inhibin B and an increase in activin A may contribute in part to the rise in follicular phase follicle-stimulating hormone of aging cycling women. J Clin Endocrinol Metab 1998;83:3302–3307.

31 Santoro N, Adel T, Skurnick JH: Decreased inhibin tone and increased activin A secretion characterize reproductive aging in women. Fertil Steril 1999; 71:658–662.

32 Welt CK, McNicholl DJ, Taylor AE, Hall JE: Female reproductive aging is marked by decreased secretion of dimeric inhibin. J Clin Endocrinol Metab 1999;84:105–111.

33 Danforth DR, Arbogast LK, Mroueh J, et al: Dimeric inhibin: a direct marker of ovarian aging. Fertil Steril 1998;70:119–123.

34 Burger HG, Groome NP, Robertson DM: Both inhibin A and B respond to exogenous follicle-stimulating hormone in the follicular phase of the human menstrual cycle. J Clin Endocrinol Metab 1998;83:4167–4169.

35 Tong S, Wallace EM, Burger HG: Inhibins and activins: clinical advances in reproductive medicine. Clin Endocrinol (Oxf) 2003;58:115–127.

36 Lenton EA, Sexton L, Lee S, Cooke ID: Progressive changes in LH and FSH and LH: FSH ratio in women throughout reproductive life. Maturitas 1988;10:35–43.

37 Faddy MJ, Gosden RG, Gougeon A, Richardson SJ, Nelson JF: Accelerated disappearance of ovarian follicles in mid-life: implications for forecasting menopause. Hum Reprod 1992;7:1342–1346.

38 Faddy MJ, Gosden RG: A mathematical model of follicle dynamics in the human ovary. Hum Reprod 1995;10:770–775.

39 Flaws JA, Langenberg P, Babus JK, Hirshfield AN, Sharara FI: Ovarian volume and antral follicle counts as indicators of menopausal status. Menopause 2001;8:175–180.

40 Hansen KR, Morris JL, Thyer AC, Soules MR: Reproductive aging and variability in the ovarian antral follicle count: application in the clinical setting. Fertil Steril 2003;80:577–583.

41 Scheffer GJ, Broekmans FJ, Looman CW, et al: The number of antral follicles in normal women with proven fertility is the best reflection of reproductive age. Hum Reprod 2003;18:700–706.

42 Burger HG, Mamers P, Groome N: Inhibins A and B are regulated differentially in the early post-partum period. Clin Endocrinol (Oxf) 2000;53:149–153.

43 Klein NA, Battaglia DE, Woodruff TK, et al: Ovarian follicular concentrations of activin, follistatin, inhibin, insulin-like growth factor I (IGF-I), IGF-II, IGF-binding protein-2 (IGFBP-2), IGFBP-3, and vascular endothelial growth factor in spontaneous menstrual cycles of normal women of advanced reproductive age. J Clin Endocrinol Metab 2000; 85:4520–4525.

44 Klein NA, Battaglia DE, Fujimoto VY, Davis GS, Bremner WJ, Soules MR: Reproductive aging: accelerated ovarian follicular development associated with a monotropic follicle-stimulating hormone rise in normal older women. J Clin Endocrinol Metab 1996;81:1038–1045.

45 Metcalf MG: Incidence of ovulatory cycles in women approaching the menopause. J Biosocial Sci 1979;11:39–48.

46 Landgren BM, Collins A, Csemiczky G, Burger HG, Baksheev L, Robertson DM: Menopause transition: annual changes in serum hormonal patterns over the menstrual cycle in women during a nine-year period prior to menopause. J Clin Endocrinol Metab 2004;89:2763–2769.

47 Batista MC, Cartledge TP, Zellmer AW, et al: Effects of aging on menstrual cycle hormones and endometrial maturation. Fertil Steril 1995;64:492–499.

48 Santoro N, Crawford SL, Lasley WL, et al: Factors related to declining luteal function in women during the menopausal transition. J Clin Endocrinol Metab 2008; in press.

49 Skurnick J, Weiss G, Goldsmith LT, Santoro N: Longitudinal changes in hypothalamic and ovarian fuction in perimenopausal women with anovulatory cycles: relationship with vasomotor symptoms. Fert Steril 2008; in press.

50 Soules MR, Sherman S, Parrott E, et al: Executive summary: Stages of Reproductive Aging Workshop (STRAW). Fertil Steril 2001;76:874–878.

51 Metcalf MG, Donald RA, Livesey JH: Pituitary-ovarian function before, during and after the menopause: a longitudinal study. Clin Endocrinol (Oxf) 1982;17:489–494.

52 Ferrell RJ, Simon JA, Pincus SM, et al: The length of perimenopausal menstrual cycles increases later and to a greater degree than previously reported. Fertil Steril 2006;86:619–624.

53 DeWaay DJ, Syrop CH, Nygaard IE, Davis WA, Van Voorhis BJ: Natural history of uterine polyps and leiomyomata. Obstet Gynecol 2002;100:3–7.

54 Santoro N, Brockwell S, Johnston J, et al: Helping midlife women predict the onset of the final menses: SWAN, the Study of Women's Health Across the Nation. Menopause 2007;14:415–424.

55 Schoenbaum EE, Hartel D, Lo Y, et al: HIV infection, drug use, and onset of natural menopause. Clin Infect Dis 2005;41:1517–1524.

56 Luborsky JL, Meyer P, Sowers MF, Gold EB, Santoro N: Premature menopause in a multi-ethnic population study of the menopause transition. Hum Reprod 2003;18:199–206.

57 Cramer DW, Barbieri RL, Xu H, Reichardt JK: Determinants of basal follicle-stimulating hormone levels in premenopausal women. J Clin Endocrinol Metab 1994;79:1105–1109.

58 Barbieri RL, Gao X, Xu H, Cramer DW: Effects of previous use of oral contraceptives on early follicular phase follicle-stimulating hormone. Fertil Steril 1995;64:689–692.

59 Sternfeld B, Bhat AK, Wang H, Sharp T, Quesenberry CP Jr: Menopause, physical activity, and body composition/fat distribution in midlife women. Medicine and science in sports and exercise 2005; 37:1195–1202.

60 Do KA, Treloar SA, Pandeya N, et al: Predictive factors of age at menopause in a large Australian twin study. Hum Biol 1998;70:1073–1091.

61 Treloar SA, Do KA, Martin NG: Genetic influences on the age at menopause. Lancet 1998;352:1084–1085.

62 Gosden RG, Treloar SA, Martin NG, et al: Prevalence of premature ovarian failure in monozygotic and dizygotic twins. Hum Reprod 2007;22:610–615.

63 Weel AE, Uitterlinden AG, Westendorp IC, et al: Estrogen receptor polymorphism predicts the onset of natural and surgical menopause. J Clin Endocrinol Metab 1999;84:3146–3150.

64 Toner JP: Ovarian reserve, female age and the chance for successful pregnancy. Minerva Ginecol 2003;55:399–406.

65 Seifer DB, Lambert-Messerlian G, Hogan JW, Gardiner AC, Blazar AS, Berk CA: Day 3 serum inhibin-B is predictive of assisted reproductive technologies outcome. Fertil Steril 1997;67:110–114.

66 Corson SL, Gutmann J, Batzer FR, Wallace H, Klein N, Soules MR: Inhibin-B as a test of ovarian reserve for infertile women. Hum Reprod 1999;14:2818–2821.

67 Hofmann GE, Danforth DR, Seifer DB: Inhibin-B: the physiologic basis of the clomiphene citrate challenge test for ovarian reserve screening. Fertil Steril 1998;69:474–477.

68 Ravhon A, Lavery S, Michael S, et al: Dynamic assays of inhibin B and oestradiol following buserelin acetate administration as predictors of ovarian response in IVF. Hum Reprod 2000;15:2297–2301.

69 Dzik A, Lambert-Messerlian G, Izzo VM, Soares JB, Pinotti JA, Seifer DB: Inhibin B response to EFORT is associated with the outcome of oocyte retrieval in the subsequent in vitro fertilization cycle. Fertil Steril 2000;74:1114–1117.

70 Tsepelidis S, Devreker F, Demeestere I, Flahaut A, Gervy C, Englert Y: Stable serum levels of anti-Mullerian hormone during the menstrual cycle: a prospective study in normo-ovulatory women. Hum Reprod 2007;22:1837–1840.

71 van Rooij IA, Broekmans FJ, te Velde ER, et al: Serum anti-Mullerian hormone levels: a novel measure of ovarian reserve. Hum Reprod 2002;17:3065–3071.

72 Visser JA, de Jong FH, Laven JS, Themmen AP: Anti-Mullerian hormone: a new marker for ovarian function. Reproduction 2006;131:1–9.

73 Santoro N, Lo Y, Moskaleva G, et al: Factors affecting reproductive hormones in HIV-infected, substance-using middle-aged women. Menopause 2007;14:859–865.

74 Frattarelli JL, Levi AJ, Miller BT, Segars JH: A prospective assessment of the predictive value of basal antral follicles in in vitro fertilization cycles. Fertil Steril 2003;80:350–355.

75 Golden TR, Hinerfeld DA, Melov S: Oxidative stress and aging: beyond correlation. Aging Cell 2002; 1:117–123.

76 Droge W: Oxidative stress and aging. Adv Exp Med Biol 2003;543:191–200.

77 Devi SA, Kiran TR: Regional responses in antioxidant system to exercise training and dietary vitamin E in aging rat brain. Neurobiol Aging 2004;25:501–508.

78 Heilbronn LK, Ravussin E: Calorie restriction and aging: review of the literature and implications for studies in humans. Am J Clin Nutr 2003;78:361–369.

79 Lane N: A unifying view of ageing and disease: the double-agent theory. J Theor Biol 2003;225:531–540.

80 Luczaj W, Waszkiewicz E, Skrzydlewska E, Roszkowska-Jakimiec W: Green tea protection against age-dependent ethanol-induced oxidative stress. J Toxicol Environ Health A 2004;67:595–606.

81 Van Remmen H, Ikeno Y, Hamilton M, et al: Lifelong reduction in MnSOD activity results in increased DNA damage and higher incidence of cancer but does not accelerate aging. Physiol Genom 2003;16:29–37.

82 Liu L, Keefe DL: Ageing-associated aberration in meiosis of oocytes from senescence-accelerated mice. Hum Reprod 2002;17:2678–2685.

83 Naeye RL: Maternal age, obstetric complications, and the outcome of pregnancy. Obstet Gynecol 1983;61:210–216.

84 Guzick DS, Talbott EO, Sutton-Tyrrell K, Herzog HC, Kuller LH, Wolfson SK Jr: Carotid atherosclerosis in women with polycystic ovary syndrome: initial results from a case-control study. Am J Obstet Gynecol 1996;174:1224–1229; discussion 9–32.

85 Ostberg JE, Donald AE, Halcox JP, Storry C, McCarthy C, Conway GS: Vasculopathy in Turner syndrome: arterial dilatation and intimal thickening without endothelial dysfunction. J Clin Endocrinol Metab 2005;90:5161–5166.

86 Seeman TE, McEwen BS, Rowe JW, Singer BH: Allostatic load as a marker of cumulative biological risk: MacArthur studies of successful aging. Proc Natl Acad Sci U S A 2001;98:4770–4775.

87 McEwen BS: Stress, adaptation, and disease: allostasis and allostatic load. Ann NY Acad Sci 1998; 840:33–44.

88 Kirkwood TB, Shanley DP: Food restriction, evolution and ageing. Mech Age Dev 2005;126:1011–1016.

89 Barzilai N, Atzmon G, Derby CA, Bauman JM, Lipton RB: A genotype of exceptional longevity is associated with preservation of cognitive function. Neurology 2006;67:2170–2175.

90 Atzmon G, Schechter C, Greiner W, Davidson D, Rennert G, Barzilai N: Clinical phenotype of families with longevity. J Am Geriatr Soc 2004;52:274–277.

91 Barzilai N, Gabriely I, Gabriely M, Iankowitz N, Sorkin JD: Offspring of centenarians have a favorable lipid profile. J Am Geriatr Soc 2001;49:76–79.

92 Pal L, Santoro N: Premature ovarian failure: discordance between somatic and reproductive aging. Ageing Res Rev 2002;1:413–423.

93 Battaglia DE, Goodwin P, Klein NA, Soules MR: Influence of maternal age on meiotic spindle assembly in oocytes from naturally cycling women. Hum Reprod 1996;11:2217–2222.

94 Liu L, Franco S, Spyropoulos B, Moens PB, Blasco MA, Keefe DL: Irregular telomeres impair meiotic synapsis and recombination in mice. Proc Natl Acad Sci USA 2004;101:6496–6501.

95 Weiss G, Skurnick JH, Goldsmith LT, Santoro NF, Park SJ: Menopause and hypothalamic-pituitary sensitivity to estrogen. JAMA 2004;292:2991–2996.

96 Scarbrough K, Wise PM: Diurnal rhythmicity of norepinephrine activity associated with the estradiol-stimulated luteinizing hormone surge: effect of age and long-term ovariectomy on hemispheric asymmetry. Biol Reprod 1991;44:769–775.

97 Santoro N, Banwell T, Tortoriello D, Lieman H, Adel T, Skurnick J: Effects of aging and gonadal failure on the hypothalamic-pituitary axis in women. Am J Obstet Gynecol 1998;178:732–741.

98 Morley JE: The metabolic syndrome and aging. J Gerontol [A] 2004;59:139–142.

99 Hoffman AR, Ceda GP: Should we treat the somatopause? J Endocrinol Invest 1999;22:4–6.

100 Labrie F, Belanger A, Cusan L, Gomez JL, Candas B: Marked decline in serum concentrations of adrenal C19 sex steroid precursors and conjugated androgen metabolites during aging. J Clin Endocrinol Metab 1997;82:2396–2402.

101 Purnell JQ, Brandon DD, Isabelle LM, Loriaux DL, Samuels MH: Association of 24-hour cortisol production rates, cortisol-binding globulin, and plasma-free cortisol levels with body composition, leptin levels, and aging in adult men and women. J Clin Endocrinol Metab 2004;89:281–287.

102 Vgontzas AN, Zoumakis M, Bixler EO, et al: Impaired nighttime sleep in healthy old versus young adults is associated with elevated plasma interleukin-6 and cortisol levels: physiologic and therapeutic implications. J Clin Endocrinol Metab 2003; 88:2087–2095.

103 Carr MC: The emergence of the metabolic syndrome with menopause. J Clin Endocrinol Metab 2003;88:2404–2411.

104 Mogul HR, Weinstein BI, Mogul DB, et al: Syndrome W: a new model of hyperinsulinemia, hypertension and midlife weight gain in healthy women with normal glucose tolerance. Heart Disease 2002;4:78–85.

105 Snowdon DA, Kane RL, Beeson WL, et al: Is early natural menopause a biologic marker of health and aging? Am J Publ Health 1989;79:709–714.

106 Anderson GL, Limacher M, Assaf AR, et al: Effects of conjugated equine estrogen in postmenopausal women with hysterectomy: the Women's Health Initiative randomized controlled trial. JAMA 2004; 291:1701–1712.

107 Rossouw JE, Anderson GL, Prentice RL, et al: Risks and benefits of estrogen plus progestin in healthy postmenopausal women: principal results From the Women's Health Initiative randomized controlled trial. JAMA 2002;288:321–333.

108 Sowers M, Jannausch ML, Gross M, et al: Performance-based physical functioning in African-American and Caucasian women at midlife: considering body composition, quadriceps strength, and knee osteoarthritis. Am J Epidemiol 2006;163:950–958.

109 Bromberger JT, Assmann SF, Avis NE, Schocken M, Kravitz HM, Cordal A: Persistent mood symptoms in a multiethnic community cohort of pre- and perimenopausal women. Am J Epidemiol 2003;158:347–356.

110 Freeman EW, Sammel MD, Liu L, Gracia CR, Nelson DB, Hollander L: Hormones and menopausal status as predictors of depression in women in transition to menopause. Arch Gen Psychiatry 2004;61:62–70.

111 Dennerstein L, Dudley EC, Hopper JL, Guthrie JR, Burger HG: A prospective population-based study of menopausal symptoms. Obstet Gynecol 2000; 96:351–358.

112 Gold EB, Sternfeld B, Kelsey JL, et al: Relation of demographic and lifestyle factors to symptoms in a multi-racial/ethnic population of women 40–55 years of age. Am J Epidemiol 2000;152:463–473.

113 de Vet A, Laven JS, de Jong FH, Themmen AP, Fauser BC: Antimullerian hormone serum levels: a putative marker for ovarian aging. Fertil Steril 2002;77:357–362.

Nanette Santoro
Division of Reproductive, Endocrinology, Albert Einstein College of Medicine
1300 Morris Park Avenue, Mazer 314
Bronx, NY 10461 (USA)
Tel. +1 718 430 3152, Fax +1 718 430 8586, E-Mail glicktoro@aol.com

Soares CN, Warren M (eds): The Menopausal Transition. Interface between Gynecology and Psychiatry.
Key Issues in Mental Health. Basel, Karger, 2009, vol 175, pp 18–40

Sexuality during Menopause: Deconstructing the Myths

Anita H. Clayton · David V. Hamilton

Department of Psychiatry and Neurobehavioral Sciences, University of Virginia Health
System, Charlottesville, Va., USA

Abstract

The menopausal transition is associated with significant psychosocial changes and dramatic alterations in the internal hormonal milieu, which may be associated with negative affects on sexual interest and activity. While one-third of women report sexual activity for nonsexual reasons, two-thirds
maintain sexual interest and satisfaction through the menopausal transition. Although the percentage of women with low desire increases with age, because associated distress decreases, the prevalence of hypoactive sexual desire disorder (diminished desire plus distress) remains unchanged
across the lifespan, affecting 10–15% of women. Problems with arousal and orgasmic dysfunction
are associated with declining levels of sex steroids, and may also be associated with partner sexual
or relationship problems, absence of a partner, medical or psychiatric illness, and/or effects of medication. Other risk factors include surgical menopause at a young age, severe vasomotor symptoms,
socioeconomic issues, and lifestyle factors such as smoking and alcohol use. Interventions for a
decline in sexual interest or function at midlife include lubricants, supplementation of sex steroids
(predominately estrogen and androgens) either as a prescription or as phytoestrogens, phosphodi-
esterase-5 inhibitors, bupropion, lifestyle changes, and psychotherapy. Identifying sexual problems
in mid-life women allows for appropriate interventions to aid in re-establishing a satisfactory sex life
after menopause.   Copyright © 2009 S. Karger AG, Basel

More than 40 years have elapsed since the advent of safe, easily attainable contraception for women. The availability of reliable contraception has minimized the specter
of inevitable pregnancy as a consequence of sexual activity, and with this freedom has
come a sea change in cultural attitudes, norms, and mores about women's sexuality.
With the power to decide if sexual activity has procreation as its goal, younger women
are increasingly marrying later, delaying starting a family, and, should they choose,
taking the time to advance their education and careers.

As such, the study of postmenopausal sexuality is a relatively new area of inquiry.
Though rigorous epidemiological study of female sexuality essentially began with
Kinsey and his research staff publishing *Sexual Behavior of the Human Female* in

1953, the specific study of postmenopausal sexuality did not begin in earnest until the 1990s. As early as 1985, Sarrel and Whitehead [1] reported that a large majority of their postmenopausal patients experienced some 'psychosexual problem'. Women who had problems prior to menopause found that these problems grew worse. Most of those women who reported experiencing sexual problems, however, developed problems during the years immediately proceeding and following menopause. These problems included disorders of sexual desire, sexual response and sexual behavior.

Nature abhors a vacuum, so to fill the knowledge gap, various myths have developed around female sexuality at mid-life and beyond. These myths include: (1) Women lose all interest in sex with onset of menopause. If women continue to participate in sexual activity during the peri- and postmenopause, significant problems with arousal and orgasmic capacity develop. (2) When sexual problems develop at mid-life, there are no effective interventions available.

Let us examine the data now available regarding these beliefs.

Epidemiology

In a large (n = 2,073), questionnaire-based study done during the early 1990s, Nusbaum et al. [2] found that nearly all (i.e. 98%) of women reported having one or more sexual concerns. They found that the nature of these concerns changed during a women's lifespan. Younger women (<45 years) reported concerns related to physical or sexual abuse, safe sex, same sex issues, concerns about body image, and family planning. Although the proportion of women reporting concerns with sexual function such as lack of interest, sexual aversion, and difficulty with orgasm and intercourse were similar across the three age groups, the intensity of these concerns grew in the middle group (ages 45–55 years), and were higher still in the older group (>55 years). A higher proportion of women in the older group reported being pre-orgasmic, a term used by the authors to indicate women who had never experienced an orgasm. However, older women reported less concern about body image, which the authors attributed to either an effect of maturity, or diminished cultural pressures emphasizing physical beauty with aging [2].

Nusbaum et al. [2] also found that in all 3 age categories only 14–17% of women (difference not significant) reported that their doctor had brought up the subject of sexual function, and the majority of women had never spoken with their doctor about sex. When the topic had been raised, the patient was nearly twice as likely as the physician to have initiated the topic, regardless of age group. The majority of women in each age category believed that their physician would not be receptive to discussing their sexual concerns, either because they felt their doctor was too embarrassed or was simply not interested.

In 1995, Dennerstein et al. [3] reported the results of a large (n = 2,001) cross-sectional telephone survey of randomly selected Australian-born women between the ages of 45 and 55. The survey posed questions related to changes in sexual interest over the year prior to interview, possible reasons for any change in interest, frequency of sexual intercourse, and dyspareunia. Thirty-one percent of the women interviewed reported a decline in sexual interest, while 62% reported no change. In those women reporting decreased interest, natural menopause (rather than age) was significantly associated ($p < 0.01$), as was a feeling of decreased physical well-being ($p < 0.001$). Socioeconomic factors were also significantly associated with sexual interest: decreasing employment was associated with decline ($p < 0.01$), while 11–12 years of education were found to protect against a decline in desire ($p < 0.01$). In addition, more severe menopausal vasomotor symptoms were associated with decreased sexual interest ($p < 0.01$), as was the presence of cardiopulmonary and skeletal disease symptoms ($p < 0.001$ and 0.01, respectively). The authors make the point that these associations, while not indicative of causality, could inform the direction of future study.

The finding that socioeconomic factors play a role in postmenopausal sexuality was replicated in a large Canadian study in which 15,249 women ages 35–59 years reported on the frequency of sexual intercourse. Data were extracted from Canada's National Population Health Survey. Across this large sample, sociodemographic and lifestyle factors were the most consistent predictors of participants' frequency of sexual intercourse. Smoking was found to be the lifestyle factor with the largest negative effect size across all age groups. While alcohol use was found to be associated with higher frequency of sexual intercourse, these data are difficult to interpret, as the highest alcohol use category was 'regular drinker', which was defined as 1 or more drinks per month. This categorical definition captures both relatively intermittent social drinkers as well as those with an alcohol problem. Though the study found a lower frequency of sexual intercourse among older non-Caucasian women, this result may reflect the lack of availability of preferred partners, if women prefer partners from their own ethno-racial group (given the relative homogeneity of the Canadian population). Alternatively, this finding may represent a true cultural effect [4].

Recent studies have identified variations in the prevalence rates of sexual disorders in women that are associated with differences in ethnic and racial background. The Study of Women's health Across the Nation (SWAN) used phone and clinic-based interviews to establish the rates of sexual dysfunction in 3,167 white non-Hispanic, African-American, Hispanic, Chinese, and Japanese women, aged 42–52 years, who were not using hormones [5]. Researchers found that premenopausal women reported less pain with intercourse than perimenopausal women ($p = 0.01$), but these two groups did not differ in frequency of intercourse, desire, arousal, or physical or emotional satisfaction. Relationship factors, the perceived importance of sex, attitudes toward aging, and vaginal dryness were the variables having the greatest association across all outcomes. Controlling for sociodemographic factors such as income, amount of education and geography, significant ethnic differences were found for arousal, pain, desire and frequency of sexual intercourse. African-American women reported higher frequency of sexual intercourse than white, non-Hispanic women.

Hispanic women reported lower physical pleasure and arousal. Both Chinese and Japanese women reported more pain, less desire, and less arousal that white women, although only the difference in arousal was statistically significant.

Few studies in the United States have specifically addressed the incidence and prevalence rate of sexual dysfunction among women. In one of the few studies to address the issue, Bancroft et al. [6] found that among Caucasian and African-American women between 20 and 65 years of age who were asked about their degree of distress associated with sexual problems, 24% of women reported marked distress about their sexual relationship, their own sexuality, or both. While this study provided valuable preliminary results, it did not address whether changes in sexual function were associated with naturally or surgically postmenopausal status. Validated scales to assess either low sexual desire or distress were not utilized. Furthermore, the specific concern was not recorded, for instance, whether women experienced difficulties with desire, arousal or excitement, inability to reach orgasm, or some admixture of these. Other factors that may also affect female sexual functioning, particularly with the menopause, include sexual dysfunction in the partner, absence of a partner, and other changes in the intimate relationship. Medical and psychiatric illness and use of associated treatments (e.g. medications) increase in incidence at midlife, and may also negatively impact sexual functioning.

The primary sexual disorder associated with desire is hypoactive sexual desire disorder (HSDD). The Diagnostic and Statistical Manual for Mental Disorders, ed 4, text revision (DSM-IV-TR) states that women with low sexual desire may only be classified as having HSDD if they are experiencing personal distress resulting from their low sexual desire [7]. The National Health and Social Life Survey, a study of adult sexual behavior conducted in the United States, found that approximately one third of all women reported low sexual interest and 44% reported some kind of sexual dysfunction [8]. However, since no questions were asked about whether their low desire was distressing or problematic, these results cannot be viewed as prevalence rates for HSDD.

The two key criteria for the diagnosis of HSDD are (1) the experiencing of difficulty in the desire phase of the sexual response cycle, and (2) that this difficulty causes marked distress. Leiblum et al. [9] reported on HSDD from data collected as part of the Women's International Study of Health and Sexuality (WISHeS), employing two valid and reliable psychometric instruments to determine women with or without HSDD. In all, three validated instruments or scales were contained in the survey, including the Short Form-36 (SF-36) to assess overall health status, the Profile of Female Sexual Function (PFSF) to assess sexual desire in women, and the Personal Distress Scale (PDS) to assess distress experienced by women due to low sexual desire. The survey also asked about the frequency of sexual activity, satisfaction with sexual life, and satisfaction with partner relationships during the preceding 30 days.

The WISHeS data demonstrated that HSDD ranged in prevalence from 9% in naturally postmenopausal women to 26% in younger surgically postmenopausal women.

Surgically postmenopausal women, aged 20–49 years, reported a significantly higher prevalence than premenopausal women of similar age. No significant differences were found in the prevalence of HSDD between surgically postmenopausal women, aged 50–70 years, and naturally postmenopausal women in the same age group. For many women, in addition to emotional and psychological distress, HSDD was associated with a significantly lower sexual and partner satisfaction. HSDD was also associated with significant decrements in general health status, including aspects of mental and physical health.

Low sexual desire was associated not only with decreased arousal, orgasm, and pleasure, and reduced frequency of sexual intercourse, but was also associated with decreased relationship satisfaction. Decrements in desire and relationship satisfaction were significantly, but not strongly, correlated. However, the direction of causality could not be established from these results; that is, decreased satisfaction could cause decreased sexual desire, or vice versa. An incontrovertible result of the study was that relationship and sexual problems coexist for many women [9].

Burleson et al. [10] recently reported the results of a smaller study (n = 58) that directly explored the relationship between mood, stress, nonsexual physical affection and sexual activity in middle-aged, perimenopausal women (mean age = 47.6 years). All of these women were not lactating, pregnant, or more than a year from their last menstrual period. Daily ratings were performed by these women for 36 weeks. Physical affection or sexual behavior with a partner on 1 day significantly predicted lower experience of negative mood, higher positive mood, and lower stress on the following day. This relationship did not hold for orgasms achieved without a partner. Conversely, positive mood on 1 day predicted more physical affection and sexual activity on the next day, and fewer non-partnered orgasms. However, negative mood was not positively or negatively correlated with the next day's sexual activity. The authors concluded that these results support a bidirectional causal model, in which physical affection and sexual activity improve mood and reduce stress, and improved mood and reduced stress in turn increase the likelihood of future sexual activity and physical affection. Of note, though 24.1% of the women self-identified as being lesbian, no significant differences were found on the basis of sexual orientation.

While it is well known that mood disorders can contribute to sexual dysfunction, only recently has this interaction been studied specifically in women at midlife. In a study of 914 women aged 42–52 years, women with a history of recurrent major depressive disorder reported experiencing less frequent sexual arousal, physical pleasure, and emotional satisfaction within their current sexual relationships.

However, no difference was reported in rates of desire between women with a history of a single depressive episode, recurrent depression, or no history of depression. Despite remission of depressive symptoms, rates of decreased physical pleasure and less satisfying emotional relationships were unchanged. Recurrent depression was also associated with higher rates of self-stimulation, possibly representing an attempt to compensate for reduced physical pleasure [11].

These findings appear to be consistent across cultures. A recent study shows that Moroccan sexual dysfunction rates are similar to those found in North America, Europe, and Australia [12]. Of the 728 women sample, 29% had no education, 78% pursued no professional activity, and 58% were married. These sociodemograpic factors indicate a population much different than that of the North American, European, or Australian samples. However, 26.6% of participants reported having sexual dysfunction always or often during the 6 months prior to the study. Though HSDD was found in 18.3% of subjects, the prevalence of the disorder decreased in the postmenopausal age cohort. When asked to explain the causes of sexual dysfunction, participants reported a variety of reasons: conflict with partner (92.9%), sexual dysfunction of the partner (90%), and poor knowledge of their bodies and erogenous zones (89.1%). These rates are very similar to those reported from North American studies. However, unlike the women in Westernized cultures, 82.3% of Moroccan subjects believed their sexual dysfunction to be a consequence of sorcery.

There has been recent debate in the literature centered around theoretical models of female sexual function. Different models attempt to define the aims of female sexual function, the thought being that the motives underlying sexual activity must be understood in order to accurately describe what is meant by sexual dysfunction, with the accurate description of sexual dysfunction being essential to its treatment. Sand and Fisher [13] were the first to perform an epidemiologic study regarding which model women at midlife endorse. A random sample of 133 registered nurses, aged 25–69 years (53% >50 years), responded to a 58-item questionnaire assessing their perception of the fit of their sexual experience with one of three theoretical models. These models included: the Masters and Johnson model (i.e. having sex in order to experience sexual feelings like orgasm), the Kaplan model (i.e. sex as a way to achieve emotional intimacy), and the Basson model (i.e. sex for non-sexual reasons). The Female Sexual Function Index (FSFI) was also given to assess current sexual function, and basic health information was collected.

Women endorsing the Masters and Johnson model of sexual functioning reported engaging in sexual activity with their partner mostly because they want to have sexual feelings, sensations, excitement, and, perhaps, orgasm. For these women, the goal of sexual activity is the satisfaction of the appetitive drive of sexual desire. Those endorsing the Kaplan model engage in sexual activity mostly because they want to feel emotionally close to their partner. Sexual activity is a way of establishing, maintaining, and confirming emotional intimacy with their partner. Finally, the Basson model was endorsed by women who engage in sexual activity with their partner, even if they do not feel the sexual desire to do so, for other, nonsexual reasons such as the sexual satisfaction of her partner. Importantly, these theoretical models stipulate only the predominant originating impulse to have sexual activity on the part of the subjects. Basson model endorsers, for instance, may sometimes seek sexual contact in order to experience sexual feelings (i.e. Masters and Johnson model), though this would not be the case most of the time. Likewise, though sexual activity may occur for nonsexual reasons by a Basson model endorser, this does not exclude enjoyment of resulting sexual activity.

Sand and Fisher [13] found that the women in this study were equally likely to endorse each of these models, emphasizing the heterogeneity of women's sexual response. Women with FSFI scores in the sexually functional range were strongly associated with choosing either the Masters and Johnson model ($p < 0.0001$) or the Kaplan model ($p < 0.03$), while women who scored as sexually dysfunctional on the FSFI were most likely to choose the Basson model ($p < 0.035$). Conversely, women who endorsed the Basson model had significantly lower FSFI scores. This pattern held for the FSFI subdomain scores for all three sexual phases: desire, arousal, and orgasm.

Women who endorsed the Masters and Johnson model or the Kaplan model were more likely to report that they were very satisfied or moderately satisfied with their sexual relationship (78.8 and 80%, respectively) than women who endorsed the Basson model (56.3%, $p = 0.0001$). Finally, women who endorsed the Basson model were significantly more likely to cite being very or moderately dissatisfied with their overall sex lives (21.9%), compared with women endorsing either Masters and Johnson (6.6%) or Kaplan (13.3%, $p = 0.001$). So, when complaints of problems with desire occur at midlife, negative effects on physical and emotional sexual pleasure are also seen.

Thus, while approximately one-third of women report a decrease in sexual desire at midlife, prevalence rates of disordered desire (HSDD = diminished desire plus distress) remain stable at about 10–15% of women. Risk factors for HSDD in peri- and postmenopausal women include: surgical menopause at a young age, severe vasomotor symptoms, socioeconomic issues such as decreasing employment and limited education, and health/lifestyle factors of smoking and the use of serotonin reuptake inhibitor antidepressants. Associations, but not causality, have been found between decreased desire and relationship dissatisfaction, a sense of low physical well-being, and vaginal dryness.

Hormonal Changes during the Menopausal Transition Affecting Reproductive/ Sexual Function

Sexuality for many women at midlife is fraught with change, and may be related to psychosocial changes as children grow into adulthood and leave the home, and/or biological variations as the hormonal milieu of a woman's body changes with the menopausal transition. While many women find the cessation of menstruation a welcome relief, for some women menopause can be accompanied by symptoms that range from the merely annoying to problems so relentless and agonizing that they make everyday function itself a challenge. In order to understand the impact of menopause on sexual physiology better, a brief review of known reproductive physiology is in order.

The regulation of the hormonal cycle occurs through a complex interplay between the hypothalamus, the anterior pituitary gland, and the ovaries, the so-called HPG axis. The hypothalamus releases gonadotropin-releasing hormone (GnRH), which acts on the anterior pituitary gland to release luteinizing hormone (LH) and follicle-stimulating hormone (FSH). FSH acts on the granulosa cells of the ovary to produce estrogens and inhibin. LH stimulates ovarian theca cells to produce testosterone, some of which is converted to estrogen by the granulosa cells prior to release into circulation. In turn, estrogen acts on the anterior pituitary to inhibit release of LH, while inhibin decreases release of FSH (also at the anterior pituitary), keeping the system in balance.

Reproductive stages are classified by changes in menstrual patterns and FSH levels [14]. Prior to the onset of any changes in menstruation or symptoms of menopause, the onset of the menopausal transition begins with fluctuations in the production of GnRH, which alters the release patterns of FSH and LH. Throughout a woman's life there is a steady decline in the number of follicles present in the ovaries. Generally, sometime after age 40, the number of follicles is low enough to cause changes in menstruation. When increased release of FSH and LH can no longer compensate for the diminishing number of ovarian follicles, a number of hormonal changes emerge: androgen synthesis decreases in the theca cells (though the adrenals continue to produce a relatively small amount of androgens), estrogen levels fall, and progesterone synthesis in the corpus luteum is reduced [15]. The final menstrual period (FMP) in the naturally menopausal woman signals ovarian failure.

One year after FMP, a woman is considered to be postmenopausal. The hypothalamus and anterior pituitary continue to function throughout a woman's life, and in early menopause FSH and LH levels rise to as much as 20 times their premenopausal levels in an attempt to stimulate the production of hormones in the quiescent ovaries [16]. FSH and LH levels decline steadily after age 55, and continue to decline until age 70.

The reduction of levels of circulating hormones affects a variety of systems. Urogenital tissues including the vulva, vagina, uterus, urethra, and bladder contain a high density of estrogen receptors; withdrawal of estrogen leads to atrophy in these tissues. The uterus decreases in size and the vulva and vagina lose thickness and vascularity. Secretions from the cervix and Bartholin's glands decrease, contributing to vaginal dryness. Changes in vaginal flora lead to decreased acid production and increased pH. Vaginal atrophy and dryness may lead to pruritus, dyspareunia, and increased rates of infection. Estrogen is essential in maintaining the integrity of pelvic connective tissue, and its withdrawal during menopause can result in decreased strength in pelvic ligaments, increasing the risk of urinary stress incontinence and prolapse of both the uterus and bladder [17].

Breast tissues are also sensitive to the withdrawal of estrogen. Many postmenopausal women experience decreased tactile sensitivity in their breasts. Decreased estrogen leads to diminished fat content in the breasts, as well as decreased nipple sensitivity and erection during sexual arousal. These changes mean that greater stimulation is required to achieve sexual excitement [18].

Approximately 75% of menopausal women experience 'hot flashes': an uncomfortable sensation of sudden heat, accompanied by tachycardia, increased skin temperature, flushing, and perspiration from the face and upper body [19]. The frequency, intensity, and duration of hot flashes are highly variable, but for many women these symptoms can be extremely distressing. In approximately 50% of women who experience hot flashes, symptoms end after 5 years, but 10% of women continue to experience them for 15 years or more [20].

Neurobiology of Menopausal Sexuality

The changing hormonal milieu of the menopausal transition affects every stage of the sexual response cycle. Testosterone appears to exert the greatest influence on desire among the primary sex steroids, and increased levels of circulating, non-protein-bound testosterone may be associated with increased rates of initiation of sexual activity [21]. The neurotransmitters dopamine and serotonin may modulate testosterone function by way of the hypothalamus and associated limbic structures. Decreased levels of bioavailable testosterone may lead to symptoms of androgen insufficiency, characterized by a diminished sense of well-being or dysphoric mood, persistent and unexplained fatigue, and sexual function changes such as decreased libido, diminished sexual receptivity, and reduced pleasure [22].

Clinical detection of sexual function problems due to androgen insufficiency is complicated by a number of factors. Only bioavailable or free testosterone is able to traverse the blood-brain barrier and exert an influence on the brain structures involved in sexual function (e.g. hypothalamus, pituitary, amygdala). The majority of circulating testosterone is bound to a protein, sex hormone-binding globulin, and does not influence the central nervous system directly. Little is known about androgen effects in women relative to men, and assays used to determine the amount of both free and bound testosterone have relative ranges defined by androgen levels present in men. Furthermore, the reduction of testosterone levels during menopause is not well understood, given that androgens are produced by a number of different tissues [23].

The results of recent trials investigating the role of testosterone in postmenopausal sexual function have not yet yielded concise clinical recommendations. A recent Australian study of 1,021 women ages 18–75 years seen in a community-based setting examined the role of multiple androgens in female sexual function. Women who were taking psychiatric medications, had abnormal thyroid function, documented polycystic ovarian syndrome, or were younger than 45 years and using oral contraceptives were excluded. Outcome measures included the Profile of Female Sexual Functioning (PFSF) and serum levels of several androgens, including bound and free testosterone, androstenedione, and dehydroepiandrosterone sulfate (DHEAS). A low PFSF domain score for sexual responsiveness for women aged 45 years or older was associated with higher odds of having a serum DHEAS level below the 10th percentile for this age group (odds ratio 3.90, p = 0.004). However, the majority of women with low DHEAS levels did not have low sexual function. No single androgen level, including free testosterone, was found to be predictive of sexual functioning.

Recent studies have attempted to determine the effect of estrogen on female sexual response after menopause. Modelska et al. [24] found that lower estrogen levels in elderly, postmenopausal women were correlated with diminished sexual function. Endogenous estrogen (E_2) was sampled in postmenopausal women and compared with their levels three years later. Sexual health questionnaires were also administered at both time points. Women with E_2 levels <20 pmol/l had significantly greater discomfort and inability to relax when attempting to engage in sexual activity compared with women with levels of E_2 ≥20 pmol/l (p < 0.05). After 3 years, women with E_2 levels ≥20 pmol/l had significantly less decline in sexual enjoyment (p < 0.02), satisfaction (p < 0.02), sexual comfort (p < 0.05) and sexual feelings summary score (p = 0.001), when compared with women who had E_2 levels <20 pmol/l. While the investigators concluded that a larger sample size over a longer period was necessary to more fully power their results and quantify the relationship between E_2 and desire, they were able to show that lower levels of endogenous estrogen are associated with lower levels of sexual desire in postmenopausal women. Still, there appears to be a therapeutic window with regard to estrogen levels, as higher levels are associated with increased SHBG, thus binding more testosterone, and reducing its bioavailability.

Progesterone is associated with receptivity to partner-initiated sexual contact [25]. Progestin released by the ovaries and adrenals helps in maintaining genital structure and function [26], but can also be anti-estrogenic by down-regulating the production of estrogen. Estrogen, testosterone, and progestin influence the bioavailability and function of each other.

A number of neurotransmitters exert an influence on sexual function, as evidenced by the number of CNS medications that produce sexual side effects. Dopamine appears to mediate sexual desire and the subjective sense of arousal and the drive to continue sexual activity once it begins [27]. Norepinephrine is the principle neurotransmitter in the arousal stage of sexual response, both in the brain and the genitalia [28]. Increases in serotonergic transmission modulate dopamine and norepinephrine, diminishing the excitatory effects of both [29]. In peripheral tissues, serotonin also appears to be involved in initiating genital sexual arousal by way of effects on vascular tone and blood flow. It may also mediate uterine contractions during orgasm. In addition, serotonin can interfere with arousal via negative effects on sensation, modulation of the excitatory effects of norepinephrine and dopamine, and inhibiting the synthesis of nitric oxide (NO) [30]. Finally, serotonin inhibits orgasm in some people by stimulation of 5-HT2 receptors, as seen with SSRI-induced anorgasmia and other orgasmic dysfunction [31].

Vasocongestion of clitoral tissue during arousal is positively mediated by NO [32] and vasoactive intestinal polypeptide (VIP) [33] once sexual contact begins. However, sufficient levels of free testosterone [34] are required for NO to initiate vasocongestion with sexual stimulation. Acetylcholinergic nerve fibers innervate vascular smooth muscle in the vagina, allowing for the vaginal engorgement during arousal, and subsequent lubrication [35].

Thus, as the hormonal milieu changes across the menopausal transition, effects of sex steroids (estrogen and androgens) on the CNS and on genital structure and function diminish, leading to potential decreases in sexual desire, arousal, and orgasmic capacity. Co-morbidity of sexual problems with genitourinary conditions appears increased in peri- and postmenopausal women, and includes decreased sexual desire, problems with cognitive and genital arousal (e.g. vaginal dryness), dyspareunia, diminished frequency and intensity of orgasm, urinary incontinence, and both uterine and bladder prolapse.

Female Sexual Dysfunction and Menopause

A prevailing myth about the menopausal transition is that the end of a woman's fertility inevitably means the end of her sex life. Though many women do experience problems with sexual function, recent advances in the understanding of female sexual disorders (FSD) allow effective treatment for many of these problems. For many clinicians, the relationship between sexual functioning, age, and menopausal stage remains controversial, primarily due to older data that suggest no relationship between these factors [36]. More recent studies, however, have suggested that the prevalence rates of nearly all sexual problems increase during the menopausal transition.

Recent epidemiologic studies indicate that the prevalence of many FSDs increases with age, and that hormonal changes that occur during the menopausal transition have a negative impact on sexual function [37]. From early to late in the menopausal transition, the percentage of women with scores on the McCoy Female Sexuality Questionnaire indicating sexual dysfunction was found to rise from 42 to 88%. More severe sexual dysfunction was correlated with decreasing estrogen, but not with level of free testosterone. By the postmenopausal period, a significant decline was found in several areas of sexual response, including: sexual excitement and interest, frequency of sexual intercourse, and overall satisfaction with sexual function. Significant increases were reported in vaginal dryness and dyspareunia (i.e. pain with intercourse). Low satisfaction with partner sexual function was also significantly correlated with poor sexual function. Women with the lowest rates of sexual function were more likely to report distress about their sexuality [38].

Low sexual desire is the most frequently reported sexual complaint. In premenopausal women, low desire occurs in between 15 and 25%, while in postmenopausal women the prevalence jumps to 40–50% [39]. Lubrication problems are reported in

10–15% of premenopausal women, increasing to 25–30% of postmenopausal women. Orgasmic dysfunction is described in approximately 24% of both premenopausal and postmenopausal women. Younger women appear to have a higher rate of primary anorgasmia (i.e. having never experienced an orgasm) while postmenopausal women have a higher rate of less satisfying orgasms or secondary anogasmia associated with change in relationship or partner function, or with the use of medications, such as selective serotonin reuptake inhibitors (SSRIs) [40]. Dyspareunia is relatively uncommon in premenopausal women (approximately 5%). While the prevalence of dyspareunia is known to increase among postmenopausal women, estimations of the increased rate vary widely between 12 and 45% [41].

It should be noted, however, that not all studies report that the majority of postmenopausal women will experience a decrease in sexual desire. A 1997 Italian study found that sexual desire was diminished or very diminished in less that half (i.e. 48%) of postmenopausal women [42]. Desire was unchanged in 31% and increased in 11.5%. So, while much of the data supports an association between menopause and decreasing interest in sex, decreasing sexual desire at midlife is by no means inevitable.

The relationship between vaginal atrophy due to diminishing estrogen levels during menopause and dyspareunia is also unclear. Postmenopausal dyspareunia is usually thought to result from atrophy of the vaginal wall tissue and Bartholin's glands, leading to difficulty in lubrication and pain during sexual intercourse. However, a 1997 Danish study found that while decreasing estrogen levels during menopause were significantly associated with vaginal atrophy, there was not an association with vaginal dryness or dyspareunia [43]. This study concluded that complaints of vaginal dryness and dyspareunia should not automatically be attributed to vaginal atrophy associated with menopause. Rather, vaginal dryness and dyspareunia were thought to reflect sexual arousal problems. It should be noted, however, that this finding has not been widely accepted as disproving any relationship between vaginal atrophy, dryness, and dyspareunia. Rather, this study illustrates that our understanding of the mechanisms of these symptoms remains incomplete.

The menopausal transition appears to be associated with an increasing prevalence of FSD. However, the causal relationship between menopause and FSD remains unclear. Recent studies indicate that multiple factors influence postmenopausal sexuality: the general health and medical comorbidities of the women, changes in the levels of hormones such as estrogen, testosterone, and progestin, the sexual function of a woman's partner, a women's premenopausal sexual function, relationship factors, and a woman's expectations of her sexual functioning [44].

In order to better examine the role of relationship factors in women's sexual functioning at midlife, a recent Australian study interviewed 438 women ages 45–55 years who were still menstruating at the time of their baseline interview [45]. Eight years of longitudinal data were available for 336 of these women, none of whom underwent surgical or medication-induced menopause. A questionnaire and blood draws were performed to evaluate women for age, hormone levels (i.e. estrogen and free testosterone), menopausal status, partner status, and feelings for partner. Sexual response was found to be predicted by prior level of sexual function, change in partner status, feelings for partner, and estrogen level. Significant predictors of dyspareunia included premenopausal history of dyspareunia and, contrary to the 1997 Danish study cited above, estrogen levels. Frequency of sexual activity was predicted by prior level of sexual function and response, change in partner status, and feelings for partner. In all, prior sexual function and relationship factors were found to be more important than hormonal determinants of sexual function in perimenopausal women.

As discussed above, menopause is associated with increasing rates of stress and an increased risk of depression [12, 13]. A 2001 study investigated the association between depression and estrogen (i.e. absolute levels of estradiol, and changes in estradiol) [46]. In 309 women, aged 43–53 years at study initiation, the Center for Epidemiologic Studies-Depression (CES-D) scale was used at baseline and follow-up to determine the presence of depressive symptoms, and correlated with estradiol levels. CES-D score was not significantly associated with menopause status categories, nor was it associated with measured annual change in estradiol level ($p = 0.19$). Hot flashes were positively associated with CES-D score ($p = 0.04$), as was trouble sleeping ($p < 0.001$). However, estradiol did not have a direct effect on CES-D scores, independent of symptoms. These results were interpreted as providing strong support for the domino or symptom hypothesis, which posits that depressed mood is caused by vasomotor symptoms associated with changing estrogen levels. This study adds to the body of literature suggesting that the association between menopause and increased risk for depression may not be directly due to decreased estrogen levels. Rather, the increased prevalence of depression is most likely due to other factors, such as symptoms and sleep problems that trigger neurophysiologic changes that result in depression.

The relationship between depression and sexual dysfunction is complicated. Low libido is a common symptom in people suffering from depression. However, as we have discussed above, many of the medications used to treat depression can also contribute to sexual dysfunction. Most antidepressants have varying degrees of serotonergic activity, which can contribute to problems with all phases of the sexual response cycle. In addition, the use of antidepressant medications in postmenopausal women is further complicated by their application in the treatment of vasomotor menopausal symptoms, which themselves can contribute to poor self-image and sexual dysfunction.

Treatment

As with other cultural shifts that have resulted from the separation of sex and procreation, the standard of practice of among physicians counseling their female patients has also changed. We are expected to ask our patients about their sexual histories and provide accurate advice to help to keep them healthy and to achieve their family planning goals. However, the end of the childbearing years too often means the end of discussions about sex between patient and provider. While much has been made of how contraception has impacted women of childbearing age, few physicians have received adequate training in how to monitor a woman's sexual health through the menopausal transition and beyond, much less how to treat the sexual problems that can arise during this time.

Menopause is a time when changing hormonal levels can lead to altered physical and psychological function. Problems with sexual functioning are among the most widespread of the myriad of health issues that may arise during and after the onset of menopause. Apart from menopause itself, women at mid-life are also subject to the typical diseases of both men and women in this demographic, and sexual functioning may be affected by the pathophysiology of these disease processes, as well as their treatment.

Lubricants

Lubricants can clearly help with vaginal dryness and resulting dyspareunia, and subsequently improve orgasmic function, without any long-term safety concerns. In addition, lubricants can be used in combination with other treatments for sexual dysfunction associated with the menopausal transition. The primary objection to this intervention is displeasure with the mechanical interruption to sexual activity required for vaginal application.

Hormones

As discussed, the increase in vasomotor symptoms and FSD during menopause is due, in part, to decreasing levels of available sex hormones. The most straightforward approach to ameliorating these symptoms would seem to be providing an exogenous source for these hormones, thereby returning a woman's body to an endocrine milieu closer to its premenopausal state. A meta-analysis of 192 randomized controlled trials showed that estrogen therapy, alone or in a combination form, remains the most reliable effective therapy for relieving both the vasomotor symptoms of menopause as well as the associated sexual dysfunction [47]. However, controversy stemming from the publication of the Women's Health Initiative (WHI) findings has led to concerns that in a small percentage of women the use of hormone replacement therapy (HRT) may lead to increased risk of cardiovascular disease, cerebrovascular disease, blood clots, and breast and ovarian cancers [48–50]. Since the publication of the WHI, many clinicians and patients have determined that the increased risk of these serious data side effects is quite small for the individual patient, and in some cases the severity of postmenopausal symptoms may warrant the use of exogenous hormones as a treatment [51], at least through the perimenopause.

Many women experience the symptoms that accompany the menopausal transition as merely time-limited annoyances. However, for women who experience more severe vasomotor symptoms during the perimenopause, and into postmenopause, the experience of these symptoms mimics the symptomatology of anxiety and depressive disorders and is associated with increased scores on anxiety and depression psychometric scales [52]. Women with a history of depression are more likely to report increased severity of menopausal symptoms [53]; these data suggest a bidirectional relationship.

In order to explore this relationship, a recent study investigated the impact of hot flushes on self-concept [54]. A questionnaire was used to examine whether poor self-image during hot flushes is linked to flush distress, perceived control, flush frequency, flush chronicity, self-esteem and depression. Women who identified the experience of hot flushes as reflecting poorly on their opinion of themselves were found to identify hot flushes as severely distressing. Poor self-image was also strongly and significantly associated with depression. Severity of hot flushes, poor self-image, and depression were not statistically associated with the frequency of hot flushes. This study further illustrates the imperative to treat the symptoms of menopause in order to avoid the association between the severity of these symptoms with both depression and, as seen previously, the association between depression and sexual dysfunction in postmenopausal women.

While several trials have reported that estrogen replacement therapy (ERT) improves the desire for sex in postmenopausal women [55], there have been few randomized placebo-controlled trials in this cohort. A 1991 cross-over study investigated the effects of estrogen and progestin versus placebo on sexual desire, arousal, and mood in healthy, naturally postmenopausal women [56]. Postmenopausal women had significantly improved sexual desire and arousal during the weeks they were given hormones compared with the weeks they were given placebo. However, comparison was made between an estrogen-progesterone and estrogen-placebo group, so the lack of a pure placebo group prevents making causal conclusions. This study also did not question participants regarding frequency of intercourse or orgasm, so the affect of ERT on those factors was unknown.

A Danish study investigated the effects of long-term hormone replacement therapy (HRT) on hot flushes, sleep difficulties, sexual problems of decreased libido and dyspareunia, and blood pressure, enrolling 1,006 women ages 45–58 years [57]. HRT efficiently and significantly alleviated hot flushes, sleep problems due to hot flushes, vaginal dryness, and dyspareunia. Libido and problems with mood swings improved in the HRT group more than in the placebo group.

Not all women experience all of these postmenopausal symptoms. For women that experience vaginal atrophy and do not wish to take systemic estrogen, topical estrogen creams may be a solution. Limited randomized controlled trials have shown that low-dose local vaginal estrogen delivery is effective and well-tolerated for treating vaginal atrophy [58]. All approved vaginal estrogen products in the United States appear equally effective at the doses recommended in their labeling. In addition, pharmacodynamic differences between oral and transdermal routes [59] of estrogen administration suggest transdermal estrogen exerts minimal effects on the concentrations of total and free (i.e. bioavailable) testosterone, thyroxine, and cortisol, compared to oral estrogen. In particular, free testosterone levels were higher by 16.4% with transdermal estrogen. While this difference was statistically significant, it is not known if this effect size is large enough to recommend switching women with low libido on oral HRT to an estrogen patch.

Another recent study examined the use of progesterone cream when used in conjunction with transdermal estrogen [60]. Women applied topical progesterone 40 mg and transdermal estrogen 1 mg daily over 48 weeks, assessed at intervals of 12 weeks. Significant increases in plasma levels of progesterone and estradiol were seen after the first 12 weeks of daily transdermal application, although only low plasma progesterone levels were found (median 2.5 nmol/l) for the remainder of the study period. No change was measured at 24 and 48 weeks of combined treatment, despite reductions in menopausal symptoms. While putative natural progestin-containing creams are efficacious in the treatment of menopausal symptoms when combined with estrogen, patients should be cautioned that these creams have effects on blood levels similar to oral preparations. Though it is unlikely that topical estrogen preparations will affect serum estrogen levels to the same degree as oral HRT, perhaps due to differences in first-pass metabolism with these two routes of administration, care should still be taken to avoid using these products in women who should not be exposed to any exogenous sources of estrogen (e.g. women with a history of estrogen-receptor positive breast cancer).

Following the publication of the WHI findings, many clinicians and patients elected to withdraw HRT. A retrospective cohort study of symptom patterns following withdrawal of HRT in postmenopausal women found significant symptom emergence [61]. Of the 1,000 postmenopausal women studied, 205 (21%) had discontinued HRT due to the WHI results. Menopausal symptoms were present in 91/205 (44%) of those women, with 52/205 (25%) having vasomotor symptoms, 51/205 (25%) urogenital complaints, and 10/205 (5%) mood-related symptoms. Of the 91 symptomatic women, only 55 (60%) received therapy to relieve their symptoms. The most commonly employed treatments were topical estrogen in 33/91 (36%) women, complementary therapies (black cohosh and soy products) in 18/91 (20%) women, and venlafaxine in 13/91 (14%) women.

A testosterone patch was studied in the early 2000s for the treatment of HSDD in surgically menopausal women. A randomized, placebo-controlled study found statistically significant increases in sexual desire and frequency of satisfying sexual encounters among the group of women received the 300-µg/day dose [62]. The 150-µg/day dose showed no significant improvement in either of these outcomes, while the 450-μg/day showed no improvement in these outcomes over those achieved at the 300 mcg/d dose.

Another study assessed the efficacy and safety of the 300-μg/day testosterone patch vs. placebo during 24 weeks of administration in surgically menopausal women with HSDD on concomitant estrogen therapy [63]. In this cohort, the 300-μg/day patch was found to significantly increase satisfying sexual activity and sexual desire, and decrease personal distress. While the incidence of adverse events was similar in both groups (p > 0.05), the incidence of androgenic adverse events (e.g. acne, hirsutism) was higher in the testosterone group, though most side effects were mild.

However, the testosterone patch failed to gain FDA approval in 2004 due to concerns over long-term safety. It is approved for use in postmenopausal women in the European Union, with post-marketing data anticipated soon.

Tibolone

Tibolone is a synthetic steroid sex hormone with estrogenic, androgenic, and progestogenic effects available in the European Union. In a recent study, 48 postmenopausal women were randomized to tibolone versus estrogen-progesterone HRT for a 3-month treatment period [64]. Based on subjective qualitative scores on the Green Climacteric Scale (GCS) and McCoy Sex Scale, tibolone treatment was found to be at least as effective as HRT in improving quality of life. Tibolone was superior to HRT in perceived improvement of sexual performance, including general sexual satisfaction, sexual interest, sexual fantasies, sexual arousal and orgasm, with decreased frequency of vaginal dryness and dyspareunia.

Another study compared tibolone to transdermal estradiol (E_2)/norethisterone (NETA) (50/120 μg) in naturally postmenopausal women with FSD [65]. Self-reported Female Sexual Function Index (FSFI) scores, and Female Sexual Distress Scale (FSDS) scores were the primary outcome measures. This 24-week, multicenter, double-blind, randomized trial enrolling 403 postmenopausal women (mean age 56 years) revealed that both treatments resulted in improved overall sexual function, as determined by higher FSFI scores, increased frequency of sexual events, and reduction in sexuality-related personal distress. A significantly larger increase in FSFI total scores was seen in the tibolone group compared to the E_2/NETA group with non-significant group differences in FSDS scores, although decreases in distress were found in both groups.

Phosphodiesterase-5 (PD-5) Inhibitors

Silendafil, a PD-5 inhibitor approved for treatment of erectile dysfunction in men, was tested for treatment of female sexual arousal disorder (FSAD) in postmenopausal women; however, active treatment failed to separate from placebo in the registration trials. Some positive effects were seen in small, proof-of-concept trials in women with female orgasmic disorder (FOD) [66], but again, larger subsequent studies failed to demonstrate a significant effect. Recently, 50–100 mg/day of sildenafil was superior to placebo in improving SRI-associated arousal and orgasmic dysfunction in women, although only 20% of the women were postmenopausal [67]. Better results were seen in women with higher levels of testosterone which enhances nitric oxide function, and thyroxine. While >80% of the women complained of concomitant decreased desire at study baseline, sexual interest was unaffected by sildenafil treatment, despite improvements in orgasmic function.

Antidepressant Treatments

While SSRI antidepressants are effective for the treatment of depression and vaso-motor symptoms, sexual dysfunction may worsen, particularly in postmenopausal women not on HRT. The non-SSRI antidepressant, bupropion has been found to improve sexual desire and decrease distress in nondepressed premenopausal women with hypoactive sexual desire disorder [68]. Bupropion is a noradrenergic-dopamin-ergic reuptake inhibitor and its action on these two neurotransmitters may improve sexual desire, arousal, and orgasm. Unlike other antidepressants currently available, bupropion lacks any appreciable serotonergic activity, which may explain its absence of negative effects on sexual function. In an open-label study investigating the effects of bupropion XL on depressed women in the late reproductive, perimenopausal and postmenopausal stages (mean age = 49.8 years) [69], 24 participants, who met cri-teria for depression (HAM-D >14) and were not receiving hormonal contraceptives or HRT, were assessed at weekly intervals for 12 weeks. Treatment with bupropion XL was associated with reduction of symptoms of depression, as measured by the Hamilton Rating Scale for Depression (HAM-D), anxiety scores monitored using the Hamilton Anxiety Rating Scale (HAM-A), and menopausal symptoms assessed by the Green Climacteric Scale. Changes in Sexual Functioning Questionnaire scores increased from baseline, demonstrating improved sexual functioning. The largest gains in sexual functioning occurred in the first three weeks of treatment, suggesting that the effect of bupropion XL on sexual functioning may occur more quickly, and perhaps independent of its antidepressant effect.

Bupropion has been studied in women with FOD as well, with inconsistent results [70, 71].

Complimentary and Alternative Therapies

One study examined the effectiveness of soy preparations containing isoflavones in treatment of menopausal symptoms. Forty-eight women in late menopause were recruited and assigned to two groups, 24 women received 35 mg/day of isoflavones and 24 received 70 mg/day. A GCS modified with three additional symptoms (frequency of hot flash, incontinence, and vaginal dryness) was used to assess menopausal symptoms. The study showed that 70 mg/day of isoflavones was needed to significantly reduce vasomotor symptoms and to provide an earlier onset of improvement in somatic symptoms, though the reduction of symptoms in this group was modest. A low-dose group (35 mg/day) was used as a control instead of placebo to minimize dropout from the study. While a statistically significant reduction in menopausal symptoms was found in the 70-mg/day group compared to the 35-mg/day group, the clinical significance of the symptom alleviation was minimal.

Should a clinician chose to recommend plant-based estrogens to a patient, the patient should be made aware that there are no data yet to suggest that phytoestrogens convey less of a risk to their health than synthetic estrogens, although tolerability differences may exist.

Acupuncture is a CAM therapy that has been studied to improve selective estrogen receptor modulator (SERM), e.g. tamoxifen-induced climacteric symptoms. In 2002, 15 patients were enrolled in a pilot study to evaluate the safety and efficacy of acupuncture for the treatment of SERM-associated menopausal symptoms [72]. Patients were evaluated at baseline prior to treatment, and after 1, 3 and 6 months using the GCS. Anxiety, depression, somatic and vasomotor symptoms were improved by the treatment, although these improvements were not tested for statistical significance, presumably due to small cohort size. Libido was not affected. Given the effects of acupuncture purported by the study, this treatment modality may warrant further study. A larger, randomized, blinded, and placebo-controlled study would help substantiate the efficacy and safety of acupuncture in treating SERM-related menopausal symptoms without worsening sexual function.

Psychological Treatments

Psychotherapies have not been specifically evaluated in peri- and postmenopausal women. However, psychotherapy that has been demonstrated to be effective in women across the lifespan includes education and directed masturbation for primary anorgasmia, with systematic desensitization and cognitive behavioral therapy (CBT) for other aspects of sexual dysfunction.

Conclusions

Thus, while menopause may be an inevitable consequence of aging, affects on sexual functioning are not as negative as the myths suggest. Most women continue to be interested in sexual activity through the menopausal transition and beyond, and despite a convergence of factors that contributes to difficulties in arousal and orgasmic capacity, interventions are available to remedy these problems.

So, because women of the baby-boomer generation have been the first to reap the benefits of effective contraception, they have consequently developed a different understanding of their sexuality than that of previous generations. Now, women have become accustomed to thinking of their sexuality as not inextricably tied to procreation. As these women proceed through mid-life, they may find that the image of the sexless matronly grandmother does not describe them, or their sex lives. The responsibility of a competent practitioner will be to evaluate a woman's current sexual function in the context of the physical, psychological, and social factors associated with the menopausal transition, and the expectations each woman has for what counts as healthy and normal sexual functioning *for her*.

References

1 Sarrel P, Whitehead M: Sex and menopause: defining the issues. Maturitas 1985;7:217–224.
2 Nusbaum MRH, Helton MR, Ray N: The changing nature of women's sexual health concerns through the midlife years. Maturitas 2004;49:283–291.
3 Dennerstein L, Smith AMA, Morse CA, Burger H: Sexuality and the menopause. J Psychosom Obstet Gynaecol 1994;15:59–66.
4 Fraser J, Maticka-Tyndale E, Smylie L: Sexuality of Canadian women at midlife. Can J Hum Sexuality 2004;13:social science module.
5 Avis NE, Zhao X, Johannes CB, Ory M, Brockwell S, Greendale GA: Correlates of sexual function among multi-ethnic middle-aged women: results from the Study of Women's Health Across the Nation (SWAN). Menopause 2005;12:385–398.
6 Bancroft J, Loftus J, Long JS: Distress about sex: a national survey of women in heterosexual relationships. Arch Sex Behav 2003;32:193–208.
7 American Psychiatry Association: Diagnostic and Statistical Manual of Mental Disorders, ed 4. Washington, American Psychiatric Association, 1994.
8 Laumann EO, Paik A, Rosen RC: Sexual dysfunction in the United States: prevalence and predictors. JAMA 1999;281:537–544.
9 Leiblum SR, Koochaki PE, Rodenberg CA, Barton I, Rosen R: Sexual desire disorder in postmenopausal women: US results from the Women's International Study of Health and Sexuality (WISHeS). Menopause 2006;13:46–56.
10 Burleson MH, Trevathan WR, Todd M: In the mood for love or vice versa? Exploring the relations among sexual activity, physical affection, affect, and stress in the daily lives of mid-aged women. Arch Sex Behav 2007;36:357–368.
11 Cyranowski JM, Bromberger J, Youk A, Matthews K, Kravitz HM, Powell LH: Lifetime depression history and sexual function in women at midlife. Arch Sex Behav 2004;33,6:539–548.
12 Kadri N, Mchichi Alami KH, Mchakra Tahiri S: Sexual dysfunction in women: population-based epidemiological study. Arch Womens Mental Health 2002;5:59–63.
13 Sand M, Fisher WA: Women's endorsement of models of female sexual response: the nurses' sexuality study. J Sex Med 2007;4:708–719.
14 Arroyo A, Yeh J: Understanding the menopause transition and managing its clinical challenges. Sexuality Reprod Menopause 2005;3:12–17.
15 Weismiller D: The perimenopause and menopause experience: an overview. Clin Geriatr Med 2004;20:565–570.
16 Hall J: Neuroendocrine physiology of the early and late menopause. Endocrinol Metab Clin N Am 2004;33:637–659.
17 Wilson MM: Menopause. Clin Geriatr Med 2003;19:483–506.
18 Phillips NA: Female sexual dysfunction: evaluation and treatment. Am Fam Physn 2000;62:127–136, 141–142.
19 Walsh B, Schiff I: Vasomotor flushes. Ann NY Acad Sci 1990;592:346–356.
20 Bachmann G: Vasomotor flushes in menopausal women. Am J Obstet Gynecol 1999;180:S312–S316.

21 Persky H, Lief HI, Strauss D, Miller W, O'Brien C: Plasma testosterone level and sexual behavior in couples. Arch Sex Behav 1978;7:157–175.

22 Bachmann G, Bancroft J, Braunstein G, Burger H, Davis S, Denneerstein L, Goldstein I, Guay A, Leiblum S, Lobo R, Notelovitz M, Rosen R, Sarrel P, Sherwin B, Simon J, Simpson E, Shifren J, Spark R, Traish A: Female androgen insufficiency: the Princeton consensus statement on definition, classification, and assessment. Fertil Steril 2002;77:660–665.

23 Braunstein GD: Androgen insufficiency in women: summary of critical issues. Fertil Steril 2002;77(suppl 4):S94–S99.

24 Modelska K, Litwack S, Ewing SK, Yaffe K: Endogenous estrogen levels affect sexual function in elderly post-menopausal women. Maturitas 2004; 49:124–133.

25 Frye CA, Rhodes ME, Walf AA, et al: Diverse mechanisms mediating the effects of steroid hormones on brain and behavior (abstract). Scientific abstracts of the 40th American College of Neuropsychopharmacology Annual Meeting. Waikoloa, Hawaii, 2001, p 38.

26 Munarriz R, Kim NN, Goldstein I, Traish A: Biology of female sexual function. Urol Clin N Am 2002;29:685–693.

27 Hull EM, Eaton RC, Moses, Lorrain DS: Copulation increases dopamine activity in the medial preoptic area of male rats. Life Sci 1993;52:935–940.

28 Segraves RT: Effects of psychotropic drugs on human erection and ejaculation. Arch Gen Psychiatry 1989;46:275–284.

29 Done CJ, Sharp T: Evidence that 5-HT2 receptor activation decreases noradrenaline release in rat hippocampus in vivo. Br J Pharmacol 1992;107:240–245.

30 Frolich PF, Meston CM: Evidence that serotonin affects female sexual functioning via peripheral mechanisms. Physiol Behav 2000;71:383–933.

31 Watson NV, Gorzalka BB: Concurrent wet dog shaking and inhibition of male rat copulation after ventromedial brainstem injection of the 5-HT2 agonist DOI. Neurosci Lett 1992;141:25–29.

32 D'Amati G, di Gioia CRT, Bologna M, Giordano D, Giorgi M, Dolci S, Jannini E: Type 5 phosphodiesterase expression in the human vagina. Urology 2002;60:191–195.

33 Palle C, Bredkajer HE, Ottesen B, Fahrenkrug J: Vasoactive intestinal polypeptide in human vaginal blood flow: comparison between transvaginal and intravenous administration. J Clin Exp Pharmacol Physiol 1990;17:61–68.

34 Marin R, Escrig A, Abreu P, Mas M: Androgen-dependent nitric oxide release in rat penis correlates with levels of constitutive nitric oxide synthetase isoenzymes. Biol Reprod 2002;61:1012–1016.

35 Giuliano F, Allard J, Compagnie S, Alexandre L, Droupy S, Bernabe J: Vaginal physiological changes in a model of sexual arousal in anesthetized rats. Am J Physiol Regul Integr Comp Physiol 2001;281: R140–R149.

36 Dennerstein L, Dudley EC, Hopper JL, Burger H: Sexuality, hormones and the menopausal transition. Maturitas 1997;26:83–93.

37 Bachmann GA, Leiblum SR: The impact of hormones on menopausal sexuality: a literature review. Menopause 2004;11:120–130.

38 Dennerstein L, Alexander JL, Kotz K: The menopause and sexual functioning: a review of the population-based studies. Ann Rev Sex Res 2003;14: 64–82.

39 Castelo-Branco C, Blumel JE, Araya H, Riquelme R, Castro G, Haya J, Gramegna G: Prevalence of sexual dysfunction in a cohort of middle-aged women: influences of menopause and hormone replacement therapy. J Obstet Gynaecol 2003;23:426–430.

40 Laumann EO, Gagnon JH, Michael RT, Michaels S: The Social Organization of Sexuality: Sexual Practices in the United States. Chicago, University of Chicago Press, 1994.

41 Gregersen N, Jensen PT, Giraldi AGE: Sexual dysfunction in the peri- and postmenopause: status of incidence, pharmacological treatment and possible risks. A secondary publication. Dan Med Bul 2006; 53:349–353.

42 Pisani G, Facioni L, Fiorani F, Pisani G: Psychosexual problems in menopause (in Italian). Min Ginecol 1998;50:77–81.

43 Laan E, van Lunsen RH: Hormones and sexuality in postmenopausal women: a psychophysiological study. J Psychosom Obstet Gynecol 1997;18:126–133.

44 Dennerstein L, Dudley E, Burger H: Are changes in sexual functioning during midlife due to aging or menopause? Fertil Steril 2001;76:456–460.

45 Dennerstein L, Lehert P, Burger H: The relative effects of hormones and relationship factors on sexual function of women through the natural menopausal transition. Fertil Steril 2005;84:174–180.

46 Avis NE, Crawford S, Stellato R, Longcope C: Longitudinal study of hormone levels and depression among women transitioning through menopause. Climacteric 2001;4:243–249.

47 Nelson H, Haney H, Miller J, Nedrow A, Nicolaidis C, Vesco K, Walker M, Bougatsos C, Nygren P: Management of menopause-related symptoms: Summary [Evidence Rep Technology Assessment No. 120, AHQR Publ. No. 05-E016–1], Rockville, Agency for Healthcare Research and Quality as cited by Petersen M: Menopause and Sexuality; in Tepper MS, Owens AF (eds): Sexual Health. Westport, Praeger Press, 2007.

48 Rossouw JE, Prentice RL, Manson JE, Wu L, Barad D, Barnabel VM, Ko M, LaCroix AZ, Margolis KL, Stefanick ML: Postmenopausal hormone therapy and risk of cardiovascular disease by age and years since menopause. JAMA 2007;297:1465–1477.

49 Wassertheil-Smoller S, Hendrix SL, Limacher M, Heiss G, Kooperberg C, Baird A, Kotchen T, Curb JD, Black H, Rossouw JE, Aragaki A, Safford M, Stein E, Laowattana S, Mysiw WJ, WHI Investigators: Effect of estrogen plus progestin on stroke in postmenopausal women. The Women's Health Initiative: a randomized trial. JAMA 2003;289:2673–2684.

50 Rossouw JE, Anderson GL, Prentice RL, LaCroix, AZ, Kiiperberg C, Stefanick ML, Jackson RD, Beresford SA, Howard BV, Johnson KC, Kotchen JM, Ockene J, Writing Group for the Women's Health Initiative Investigators: Risks and benefits of estrogen plus progestin in healthy postmenopausal women: principal results From the Women's Health Initiative randomized controlled trial. JAMA 2002; 288:321–333.

51 Dennerstein G: Re: Hormones down under: hormone therapy use after the Women's Health Initiative. Aust NZ J Obstet Gynaecol 2007;47:80.

52 Juang KD, Wang SJ, Lu SR, Lee SJ, Fuh JL: Hot flashes are associated with psychological symptoms of anxiety and depression in peri- and post- but not premenopausal women. Maturitas 2005;52:119–126.

53 Parry BL, Meliska CJ, Martinez LF, Basavaraj N, Zirpoli GG, Sorenson D, Maurer EL, Lopez A, Markova K, Gamst A, Wolfson T, Hauger R, Kripke DF: Menopause: neuroendocrine changes and hormone replacement therapy. J Am Med Women Assoc 2004;59:135–145.

54 Reynolds F: Exploring self-image during hot flushes using a semantic differential scale: associations between poor self-image, depression, flush frequency and flush distress. Maturitas 2002;42:201–207.

55 Modelska K, Cummings S: Female sexual dysfunction in postmenopausal women: systematic review of placebo-controlled trials Am J Obstet Gynec 2003;188:286–293.

56 Sherwin BB: The impact of different doses of estrogen and progestin on mood and sexual behavior in postmenopausal women. J Clin Endocrinol Metab 1991;72:336–343.

57 Vestergaard P, Hermann AP, Stilgren L, Tofteng CL, Sorensen OH, Eiken P, Nielsen SP, Mosekilde L: Effects of 5 years of hormonal replacement therapy on menopausal symptoms and blood pressure: a randomised controlled study. Maturitas 2003;46:123–132.

58 North American Menopause Society: The role of local vaginal estrogen for treatment of vaginal atrophy in postmenopausal women: 2007 position statement of The North American Menopause Society. Menopause 2007;14:355–369.

59 Shifren JL, Desindes S, McIlwain M, eDoros G, Mazer NA: A randomized, open-label, crossover study comparing the effects of oral versus transdermal estrogen therapy on serum androgens, thyroid hormones, and adrenal hormones in naturally menopausal women. Menopause 2007;14:985–994.

60 Vashisht A, Wadsworth F, Carey A, Carey B, Studd J: A study to look at hormonal absorption of progesterone cream used in conjunction with transdermal estrogen. Gyn Endo 2005;21:101–105.

61 Ness J, Aronow WS, Beck G: Menopausal symptoms after cessation of hormone replacement therapy. Maturitas 2006;53:356–361.

62 Braunstein GD, Sundwall DA, Katz M, Shifren JL, Buster JE, Simon JA, Bachman G, Aguirre OA, Lucas JD, Rodenberg C, Buch A, Watts NB: Safety and efficacy of a testosterone patch for the treatment of hypoactive sexual desire disorder in surgically menopausal women: a randomized, placebo-controlled trial. Arch Intern Med 2005;165: 1582–1589.

63 Buster JE, Kingsberg SA, Aguirre O, Brown C, Breaux JG, Buch A, Rodenberg CA, Wekselman K, Casson P: Testosterone patch for low sexual desire in surgically menopausal women: a randomized trial. Obstet Gynecol 2005;105:944–952.

64 Wu MH, Pan HA, Wang ST, Hsu CC, Chang FM, Huang KE: Quality of life and sexuality changes in postmenopausal women receiving tibolone therapy. Climacteric 2001;4:314–319.

65 Nijland EA, Weijmar Schultz WC, Nathorst-Boos J, Helmond FA, Van Lunsen RH, Palacios S, Norman RJ, Mulder RJ, Davis SR, LISA study Investigators: Tibolone and transdermal E_2/NETA for the treatment of female sexual dysfunction in naturally menopausal women: results of a randomized active-controlled trial. J Sex Med 2008;5:646–656.

66 Shields KM, Hrometz SL: Use of sildenafil for female sexual dysfunction. Ann Pharmacother 2006;40:931–934.

67 Nurnberg HG, Hensley PL, Heiman JR, Croft HA, Debattista C, Paine S: Sildenafil treatment of women with antidepressant-associated sexual dysfunction: a randomized controlled trial. JAMA 2008;300:395–404.

68 Segraves RT, Croft H, Kavoussi R, Ascher JA, Batey SR, Foster VJ, Bolden-Watson C, Metz A: Bupropion sustained release (SR) for the treatment of hypoactive sexual desire disorder (HSDD) in nondepressed women. J Sex Martal Ther 2001;27:303–316.

69 Clayton AH, McGarvey EL, Dameron ZC, Dell RB, Bukenya DB: Bupropion XL in the menopausal transition: Effect on mood, anxiety and menopausal symptoms. 19th Annual US Psychiatric and Mental Health Congress, 2006.

70 Modell JG, May RS, Katholi CR: Effect of bupropion-SR on orgasmic dysfunction in nondepressed subjects: a pilot study. J Sex Marital Ther 2000;26:231–240.

71 Segraves RT, Clayton AH, Croft H, Wolf A, Segraves K: A multicenter, double-blind, placebo-controlled study of bupropion XL in females with orgasm disorder. Abstracts of the 19th Annual US Psychiatric and Mental Health Congress, 2006.

72 Porzio G, Trapasso T, Martelli S, Sallusti E, Piccone C, Mattei A, DiStanislao C, Ficorella C, Marchetti P: Acupuncture in the treatment of menopause-related symptoms in women taking tamoxifen. Tumori 2002;88:128–130.

Anita H. Clayton, MD
University of Virginia, Department of Psychiatry and Neurobehavioral Sciences
2955 Ivy Rd, Northridge Suite 210
Charlottesville, VA 22903 (USA)
Tel. +1 434 243 4646, Fax +1 434 243 4743, E-Mail ahc8v@virginia.edu

Soares CN, Warren M (eds): The Menopausal Transition. Interface between Gynecology and Psychiatry.
Key Issues in Mental Health. Basel, Karger, 2009, vol 175, pp 41–49

Cultural and Ethnic Influences on the Menopause Transition

Johannes Bitzer · Judith Alder

Division of Psychosomatic Obstetrics and Gynecology and Sexual Medicine, Department of Obstetrics and
Gynecology, University Hospitals Basel, Basel, Switzerland

Abstract

In a meta-analysis of menopausal symptoms, the most universally reported symptoms were vaginal
dryness and other urogenital symptoms like urgency, bladder pain and incontinence. Vasomotor
symptoms were reported less consistently in different cultures. Depression, sexual dysfunction and
sleep disturbances were not commonly described across cultures. It is obvious that biological and
sociocultural factors interact during the menopausal transition in the individual woman and modulate her experience of symptoms. In any culture-sensitive care for menopausal women, physicians
should be open and aware of three major culturally determined concepts: the body in health and
disease, age and aging, and menstruation and cessation of menstruation. Especially the concept
about the body in health and disease with beliefs about the optimal shape and size of the body,
including clothing and decoration of the surface, beliefs about the boundaries of the body, about
the body's inner structure and about how the body functions are very important to understand and
to integrate this understanding. For practical purposes, health professionals should: assess the woman's individual experience of physical and psychological changes; encourage the narrative of symptoms to understand the individual priorities, subjective underpinnings and interpretations; listen to
her beliefs about her body in health and disease and give a respectful feed back about your understanding of the patients' concepts; introduce the biomedical model as one possible model of understanding the changes experiences; try to find similarities between the patients' concepts and the
biomedical model; try to bring together biological, psychological and sociocultural factors contributing to the symptoms; offer different treatment options from different concepts, and encourage
shared decision-making about the individual treatment in which the physician's role is to give information which is then evaluated by the patient according to her values and priorities.

Although menopause is a biological process which normally affects all women reach-
ing a certain age most of our knowledge about physical and psychological symptoms,
endocrine changes and therapeutic interventions derives from clinical samples of
white women. It is important to be aware of the limitations of this type of knowledge
due to some methodological pitfalls:

(1) Selection bias: The menopausal transition process in white middle-class women described as a specific endocrine, biomedical phenomenon may not be representative for the total female population, therefore the results obtained may be profoundly biased and lack external validity. There may be ethnic and sociocultural factors that have an influence on this transition process with variation in the age of onset and the dynamics of this process.

(2) Reporting bias: The reporting of symptoms during the menopausal transition may be influenced to an unknown degree by sociocultural factors like health and illness beliefs, social desirability, gender role stereotypes, etc. This makes it difficult to assume that the symptoms reported in white middle-class women describe biological and pathophysiological changes that affect women in general. Thus, symptoms can be the result of a mixture of biological processes and social construction.

It seems therefore appropriate to explore some basic questions in more detail.

Is the Age of Menopause Determined Genetically or Influenced by Sociocultural and Lifestyle Factors?

The answer to this question is not yet clear. The mean age at menopause in white women from industrialized countries is between 50 and 52 years with slight evidence of increasing age over time. The age at perimenopause is 47.5 years [1]. In some studies, African-American and Latina women have been observed to have the natural menopause about 2 years earlier than white women, despite their increased relative average body mass. According to the black women's health study, however, the average age at menopause in African-American women occurs at 49.6 years which is very close to the average for Caucasian women [2]. In Mexico City, the average age at natural menopause is 46.5 years. Among Mayan women living in Yucatan and Guatemala, it is even 2.2 years earlier [3, 4]. Asian and Caucasian women tend to be of similar age at menopause, although Thai women seem to have a lower median age at menopause (49.5 years) [5]. Filipino Malay women have been reported to have an average age at menopause of 47–48 years [6].

These differences may reflect ethnic diversity or may also be due to sociocultural, behavioral and environmental factors. Some studies indicate that women living in developing countries experience menopause several years earlier than do those living in developed countries [7, 8]. It also seems that women in urban areas have a later menopause than women in rural areas [9]. This is an indication of possible life-style factors influencing the age at which natural menopause may occur. Studies have found that alcohol abuse, cigarette smoking, nulliparity, and non-use of hormonal contraceptives are associated with earlier age at menopause [10–12]. The effect of smoking is the most consistent among all these factors; in addition, physiological and psychological stress may lead to earlier menopause. Tibetan Women living at high altitude have an earlier menopause, possibly due to altitude-induced hypoxic stress [13]. Low economic status and lack of partner or family support have also been found to alter the age of menopause possibly due to psychosocial stress [12].

To What Degree Are the Symptoms Reported during the Menopausal Transition the Result of a Uniform Biological Process or Determined by Sociocultural Concepts and Beliefs?

In a meta-analysis of menopausal symptoms, the most universally reported symptoms were vaginal dryness and other urogenital symptoms like urgency, bladder pain and incontinence.

Vasomotor symptoms were less consistently reported in the different cultures. Depression, sexual dysfunction and sleep disturbance were not commonly described across cultures. Therefore, it is plausible to admit that several possible socioculturally related concepts and health beliefs may modify and modulate the menopausal experience [14].

The Concepts of the Body in Health and Disease

In western culture, the concept of health and disease is mainly determined by the paradigm of science which states that health and disease are separate entities with specific objectively measurable characteristics. Menopause is thus an objectively measurable phenomenon characterized by the ovarian aging process which manifests itself with the cessation of menses, the incapacity to reproduce and specific hormonal markers like high FSH and low estradiol. The lack of estrogen has a measurable impact on different morphological and metabolic parameters that can be quantified (e.g. changes in metabolic parameters, bone remodeling with loss of bone density, and vascular changes). All these changes are universal in all women and thus viewed as an objective picture of what menopause is and what it means in the biomedical model. Conversely, the subjective part of the menopausal experience is assessed by using 'standardized and validated' questionnaires, formed by symptom lists. Questionnaires as part of psychometric methodology try to measure and quantify the responses to objective criteria as much as possible and to allow for 'generalization'. The implicit model is that the body is like a 'machine' that is composed of well-defined objective parts with well-defined and measurable functions. In other cultures, the concepts of the body in health and disease may be completely different.

Douglas [15] talks about 'two bodies'. An individual body self (both physical and psychological) which is acquired at birth and a social body that is needed in order to live within a particular society and cultural group. The social body provides each person with a framework for perceiving and interpreting physical and psychological experiences. Helman [16] distinguishes four major socially determined groups of beliefs about the body that modify and determine the subjective 'anatomy' and 'pathology':

- Beliefs about the optimal shape and size of the body, including clothing and decoration of the surface.
- Beliefs about the boundaries of the body.
- Beliefs about the body's inner structure.
- Beliefs about how the body functions.

To understand the culturally determined concepts about the menopausal transition, it is important to review some of the beliefs about how the body functions. In most cultures, the healthy working of the body is thought to depend on the harmonious balance between two or more elements or forces within the body. The most widespread of these theories is the humoral theory, coming from ancient China and India, but also being integrated by Hippocrates into Greek Medicine. In the Hippocratic theory, the body contained four liquids or humors: blood, phlegm, yellow bile and black bile. Health was determined by the optimal balance of these four elements and disease was understood as imbalance by excess or deficiency of one of these elements. This concept spread all over the world and is an important part of lay beliefs in much of Latin America, but also in the Islamic world and in the Ayurvedic medical tradition in India [17, 18]. The 'Latin American' version of the humoral theory is the hot-cold theory of disease. Hot and cold do not pertain to an actual body temperature but to a symbolic power contained in most substances, including food herbs and medicines. To maintain health, the body's internal 'temperature' balance must be maintained between the opposing powers of hot and cold, especially avoiding prolonged exposure to either quality. Both pregnancy and menstruation are considered to be hot states and, like other hot conditions, are treated by the ingestion of cold foods or medicines or by cold treatments such as sponging with cold water. A similar concept is found in Morocco where the emphasis is placed on two of the humors: blood and phlegm [16]. The inner workings of the body are regulated by outside influences especially diet and environment. Excess blood is seen as a feature of 'hot illness', while excess phlegm in the body characterizes a cold illness.

The ayurvedic system is also based on the humoral theory but more complex and elaborated [18]. There are five bhutas or basic elements in the universe: ether, wind, water, earth and fire. These are the basic constituents of all life, and also make up the three dosas or humors (wind, bile and phlegm). Health is a state of optimal balance of these three humors and illness results from too much or too little of one of the elements. Treatment consists again in using 'cooling' and 'heat-producing' food.

Traditional Chinese medicine [16] sees health as a harmonious balance, in this case between two contrasting cosmic principles: yin, described as dark, moist, watery and female, and yang, which is hot, dry, fiery and male. The organs of the body are either predominantly yin (such as the heart, ling, spleen, kidneys and liver) or yang (such as the intestines, stomach and gallbladder). From this conceptual background the changes of the menopausal transition can be experienced as an imbalance between hot and cold, between humoral elements due to external environmental factors coming from the nutrition, the climate or even social interaction. It is then not a matter of internal endocrine changes and the treatment tries to re-establish a balance and harmony rather substitute/replace hormone levels.

Another relevant culture-specific concept is what has been called symbolic anatomies [19]. The body is then part of a wider cosmology, linking the individual body to greater forces in the universe. Often they deal with the flow or the blockage of forces or energies and they follow a 'map of the body' which is completely different from western anatomy. In traditional Chinese medicine, the body is divided by a series of meridians or invisible channels through which chi flows – the vital energy or life force. In the tantric tradition (Hinduism and Buddhism), the chakras (or wheels) are concentrations and receptors of energy along the central axis of the body. A healthy state is thus characterized by an inhibited flow of these energies and illness is due to blockages or deviations of energy. Menopausal symptoms like hot flushes are in this model the direct experience of energy and may thus either be welcomed or interpreted as blockage of energy which should be treated by re-establishing a free flow.

Age and Aging

In Japanese language, there had been traditionally no precise term for menopause or hot flush [20]. The general term 'konenki' described the aging of women not having a relation to the cessation of menses. This shows that the global concept of aging in the Japanese tradition somehow encompasses and overrides 'minor' physical changes. In other words, the perception and especially the interpretation of body signals in this case is not the summary of a list of discrete symptoms but the result of a more globalized perception of the aging process. The cessation of menses is in this concept not a hallmark of aging but obviously of minor importance in this culture. It is interesting in this context that emotional symptoms frequently reported by 'western' women were much less frequently reported in Japanese women aged 45–55. Ex: Only 13% of Japanese women in this age group reported depressed mood compared to 35.9% of women in Massachusetts [20, 21].

The same holds true for symptoms like lack of energy or irritability, which was significantly less frequently reported by Japanese women. This could well be related to the Buddhist concept of accepting changes more stoically and the ideal of a balanced and peaceful mind which is especially attributed to the aging process. There has been some controversy with respect to the influence of nutrition, in this case the daily soy consumption in Japan, which could explain part of the difference in symptom manifestation. However, studies in Australia have shown that after the introduction of HT Australian and Japanese women experienced similar menopausal symptoms with the exception of vasomotor symptoms (fewer less severe night sweats in Japanese women) [22]. Notably, the incidence of hot flushes was the same. This would be an indication that the introduction of the biomedical approach to menopause has brought about a shift in the perception and interpretation of physical and psychological symptoms from the global aging concept to a 'symptom list' concept in which symptoms can be treated by targeted therapies.

Menstruation and Cessation of Menstruation

The social perception of menstruation varies enormously among different cultures and even within the same culture. On the one hand, menstruation is associated with impurity, poisoning, danger, vulnerability and inferiority of women, leading to social isolation and repression, and on the other, it is also a symbol of fertility, female potency and power about the reproduction of the species, something awesome and fascinating. The cessation of menses is subject to the same possible ambivalent and contradictory interpretations and attributions: postmenopausal women can be perceived as freed from impurity and the negative aspects and attribution of menstruation and can thus increase their social status and get access to social activities from which they were previously excluded. For these women, the cessation of menstruation is a positive signal and is welcomed. It seems that in many cultures this 'positive concept of menopause' prevails and leads to a lack of experience or reporting of negative physical and psychological symptoms.

The positive attribution to the cessation of menses and the elevated social status of postmenopausal women can be found in various Islamic countries, in the Indian subcontinent and in some African sub-Saharan countries. In these women, the reported rate of negative menopausal symptoms (in particular hot flushes) is very low [23].

Studies in Guatemala and Mexico among Mayan women have shown that there is no concept of menopause as the time when menses cease [24]. These women report very few hot flushes or no symptoms at all although the hormonal changes are very similar to US women. In these cultures, the social status of postmenopausal women does not change as much as in the above-mentioned regions. A possible explanation of the low reporting of symptoms is that high parity and prolonged periods of lactation-related amenorrhea may provide a desensitizing effect making the transition to menopause less likely to be noted as a 'new' or 'unknown' physical condition. This fits also in the anthropological differentiation between the concept of monochromatic time (a linear model of phases in which one follows the other measured by watches) and the polychromatic time model which is much more oriented towards the importance of interpersonal encounters and life events.

Cultural Sensitive Counseling of Menopausal Women

In current medical practice, the menopausal transition is defined by the process of ovarian aging. This basic biological fact, which is universal, is the cornerstone of the biomedical oriented 'climacteric medicine'. It establishes the basis for research into the effects of ovarian aging on the various body systems, englobing genital organs, cardiovascular system, brain functioning, bone density, etc. The results of this research are various therapeutic options for women to alleviate or modify these influences of ovarian aging on the female body.

Acknowledging the large variety of the onset, the phenomenology, the subjective experience of the menopausal transition in women in different sociocultural contexts brings about the necessity for health care providers to look at the care for menopausal women from a comprehensive biopsychosocial perspective.

The practical consequences of this perspective are numerous; the patient and the physician have to establish a common platform for an encounter which enables the menopausal woman to transmit not only her subjective experience of a specific life phase in terms of bodily and mental signals and signs, but also to give to the physician information about her beliefs regarding her body, her health and illness concepts. Only by understanding the patients' world which includes her subjective anatomy, her construction of reality and her interaction with her environment can the physician have access to her individual suffering during the menopausal transition. It may be difficult for a bio-medically trained doctor to listen to concepts so different from the paradigm she or he is trained in. The culturally determined interpretation of symptoms may look to her or him illogical, uninformed, wrong and sometimes even dangerous. This may lead the physician to impose the biomedical model on the patient by hypothesis-lead questioning leading to self-fulfilling answers. The physician may apply symptom lists and find the full picture of the climacteric syndrome in the patient and therefore he/she may think that this is a case of estrogen deficiency especially if it can be documented by hormone dysregulation. However, as long as the patient experiences her symptoms from a different cognitive and social background (humoral theory, social anatomies, cultural attributions to symptoms) patient and physician will not be able to come to a shared definition and understanding of the individual's problem and suffering. What does that mean for the practice of culture sensitive counseling of menopausal women?

Counseling and care must be provided in an interactive fashion that places the patient as a person into the center. The following steps for the physician seem to us obligatory:

(a) Assess the patient's individual experience of physical and psychological changes. Encourage the narrative of symptoms to understand the individual priorities, subjective underpinnings and interpretations.

(b) Listen to her beliefs about her body in health and disease and give a respectful feedback about your understanding of the patients' concepts.

(c) Introduce the biomedical model as one possible model of understanding the changes experiences.

(d) Try to find similarities between the patients' concepts and the biomedical model.

(e) Try to bring together biological, psychological and sociocultural factors contributing to the symptoms.

(f) Offer different treatment options from different concepts.

(g) Encourage shared decision-making about the individual treatment in which the physician's role is to give information which is then evaluated by the patient according to her values and priorities.

By applying this approach, the possible benefits of biomedical research and practice to the general and sexual health of the menopausal woman can be offered and integrated into a variety of 'alternative' or 'complementary' approaches, which may be appropriate for the individual woman in her sociocultural environment.

References

1 WHO: Report of a WHO Scientific Group. Research on the Menopause. WHO Tech Rep Ser. Geneva, World Health Organization, 1981, p 8.

2 Palmer JR, et al: Onset of natural menopause in African American women. Am J Publ Health 2003; 93:299–306.

3 Beyene Y, Martin MC: Menopausal experiences and bone density of Mayan women in Yucatan, Mexico. Am J Hum Biol 2001;13:505–511.

4 Garrido-Latorre F, et al: Age of natural menopause among women in Mexico City. Int J Gynaecol Obstet 1996;53:159–166.

5 WHO: A prospective multicenter trial of the ovulation method of natural family planning. III. Characteristics of the menstrual cycle and of the fertile phase. Fertil Steril 1983;40:773–778.

6 Boulet M: The menopause and the climacteric in seven asian countries. 6th Int Congr Menopause, Park Ridge, 1990.

7 Gonzales GF, Villena A: Age at menopause in central Andean Peruvian women. Menopause 1997; 4:32–38.

8 Wasti S, et al: Characteristics of menopause in three socioeconomic urban groups in Karachi, Pakistan. Maturitas 1993;16:61–69.

9 MacMahon B, Worcester J: Age at Menopause, United States 1960–1962. Rockville, National Center for Health Statistics, 1966, vol 11, pp 1–19.

10 Torgerson DJ, et al: Alcohol consumption and age of maternal menopause are associated with menopause onset. Maturitas 1997;26:21–25.

11 McKinlay SM, Bifano NL, McKinlay JB: Smoking and age at menopause in women. Ann Intern Med 1985;103:350–356.

12 Gold EB, et al: Factors associated with age at natural menopause in a multiethnic sample of midlife women. Am J Epidemiol 2001;153:865–874.

13 Beall CM: Ages at menopause and menarche in a high-altitude Himalayan population. Ann Hum Biol 1983;10:365–370.

14 Obermeyer CM: Menopause across cultures: a review of the evidence. Menopause 2000;7:184–192.

15 Douglas M: Natural Symbols. London, Penguin, 1973.

16 Helman C: Culture Health and Illness. London, Oxford University Press, 2007.

17 Foster G: Hippocrates' Latin American Legacy: Humoral Medicine in the World. Reading, Gordon & Breach, 1998.

18 Obeyesekere G: The theory and practice of psychological medicine in the Ayurvedic tradition. Cult Med Psychiatry 1977;1:155–181.

19 Kleinman A: Patients and Healers in the Context of Culture. Berkley, University of California Press, 1981.

20 Lock M: Encounters with aging: mythologies of menopause in Japan and North America. Berkley, University of California Press, 1993.

21 McKinlay SM, McKinlay JB: Selected studies of the menopause. J Biosoc Sci 1973;5:533–555.

22 Anderson D, et al: Menopause in Australia and Japan: effects of country of residence on menopausal status and menopausal symptoms. Climacteric 2004; 7:165–174.

23 Beyene Y: Cultural significance and physiological manifestations of menopause: a biocultural analysis. Cult Med Psychiatry 1986;10:47–71.

24 Beyenne Y: Menarche to Menopause: Reproductive Lives of Peasant Women in Two Cultures. New York, State University of New York Press, 1989.

Johannes Bitzer, MD
Division of Psychosomatic Obstetrics and Gynecology and Sexual Medicine
Department of Obstetrics and Gynecology, University Hospitals Basel
CH–Basel 4031 (Switzerland)
Tel. +41 61 265 9043, Fax +41 61 265 9035, E-Mail jbitzer@uhbs.ch

Soares CN, Warren M (eds): The Menopausal Transition. Interface between Gynecology and Psychiatry.
Key Issues in Mental Health. Basel, Karger, 2009, vol 175, pp 50–65

Nonhormonal Factors Associated with Psychiatric Morbidity during the Menopausal Transition and Midlife

Joyce T. Bromberger · Nancy F. Woods

University of Pittsburgh, Pittsburgh, Pa., USA

Abstract

This chapter describes the nonhormonal factors associated with psychiatric morbidity during the menopausal transition and early postmenopause. Multiple psychosocial and health-related factors and prior exposures are associated with risk for clinical depression, anxiety, and negative mood symptoms and syndromes in women of all ages. These include low socioeconomic status, life stressors, inadequate social support, vulnerable personality traits, medical conditions, vasomotor symptoms, psychiatric history, health history, reproductive-related factors, childhood abuse and family history and genetics. Few are specific or unique to psychiatric morbidity during the menopausal transition. Those that may be more prevalent or limiting during this period of life than prior to it include vasomotor symptoms, life stressors, and increased physical problems. The extent to which the physical and biological changes during the transition make women more vulnerable to the effects of factors such as low social support, a tendency to ruminate, or a history of childhood abuse are not known.

Copyright © 2009 S. Karger AG, Basel

Multiple non-hormonal factors are associated with psychiatric morbidity during the menopausal transition. Psychiatric morbidity includes psychiatric disorders, syndromes that do not meet clinical criteria for disorder, depressive and anxious symptoms, and general psychological distress. Because of the small number of studies that have actually assessed psychiatric disorders during the menopausal transition, we will primarily discuss symptoms, syndromes and general negative mood which have been the focus of midlife studies. Nonhormonal factors cover multiple domains that encompass experiences and conditions occurring prior to the transition and those that are proximal to or concurrent with the transition. For example, prior history includes earlier psychiatric disorders, reproductive events and conditions, childhood adversity, and prior medical events and conditions. Current domains include social and demographic factors, psychological traits, lifestyle and health behaviors, medical conditions and health-related quality of life. Social and environmental stress throughout life can have short- and long-term psychiatric sequellae. Familial and genetic factors pose a risk for psychiatric morbidity.

Depression

Clinical depression is characterized by mood, somatic, and cognitive changes and is defined by a minimum of two symptoms (minor depression) and 5 symptoms (major depression) with associated impairment in functioning for at least 2 weeks. Clinical depression also includes a low level chronic depression that is defined by at least 2 symptoms persisting at least half the time for a period of 2 years [1]. Depression is approximately twice as prevalent among women as among men [2]. The relative gender differences are consistent across cultures despite the variation by country [3]. As many as 1 in 5 women experience a depressive episode during their lives. The National Comorbidity Survey (NCS) [2], based on a probability sample of residents of the USA, excluding those institutionalized, found that lifetime prevalence of major depression was as high as 23% in middle-aged women. The NCS also reported that during a 12-month period, 10–16% of women experienced an episode of depression. In the NCS data there was an increase in first onsets among women 50–54 years old [2]. Although consistent with the theory that the menopausal transition is a time of vulnerability to major depression, the size of the sample in this age range was very small and the authors considered the results unreliable [2]. The large literature on depressive symptoms and menopause has yielded contradictory findings concerning their relationship. However, recent cross-sectional and, most importantly, longitudinal studies have reported that the risk for depressive symptoms and possibly disorder increases during the menopausal transition and early postmenopause [4–9].

Only a few studies of menopause or midlife women have evaluated clinical depression [8–10]. Two studies suggest that the risk for first onset depressive syndrome or disorder is higher during the menopausal transition than in the late reproductive period [8, 9] although a third study suggests that menopausal status per se is not associated with first onset of major depression during midlife [10]. In this study, a history of any anxiety disorder at study entry doubled the odds of an incident major depression over 7 years. To what extent a susceptibility to depressive disorder and symptoms is the result of alterations in reproductive hormones is unclear. Nevertheless, while reproductive hormone perturbations may be associated with depression, there are multiple psychosocial, lifestyle, and health-related risk factors for depression in women throughout the lifecycle.

Anxiety and Psychological Distress

Anxiety is a state of cognitive and autonomic hyperarousal that can be adaptive in stressful situations by enhancing vigilance, learning and reactivity. However, in some circumstances and individuals, anxiety may become incapacitating and counterproductive [11]. Anxiety disorders refer to a group of separate conditions characterized by an exaggerated fearfulness associated in most cases with a particular situation or concern(s) and an inability to counterregulate the stress response. They include panic disorder, agoraphobia, specific phobia, social phobia, generalized anxiety disorder, post-traumatic stress disorder, and obsessive-compulsive disorder. Anxiety disorders also affect women more than men, with 36.3% of women and 25.3% of men having a lifetime history of any anxiety disorder [12]. For people between 45 and 59 years of age prevalence of any anxiety disorder is approximately 35%. The prevalence drops to 17.7% among those 60 years of age and older [12]. For generalized anxiety disorder specifically, some studies indicate that there is an increase in its incidence for women after age 35 when prevalence rates are about 10% [13]. As noted above for depression, anxiety disorders and their lesser manifestations may be a function of social environments as well as biology.

Depression and anxiety are highly comorbid. Depression can also be conceived of as a more enduring reaction to prolonged stress with loss of normal homeostatic regulation of stress response. Further, symptoms and risk factors for some anxiety disorders, such as generalized anxiety disorder, are similar to those for depression. Thus, it is not surprising that anxiety is a prevalent comorbid condition with major depressive disorder [14]. Despite the high prevalence of anxiety disorders overall, there are no studies of these during the menopausal transition and only a small number that have assessed an anxious syndrome [15]. Rather, studies focusing on the menopausal transition assess symptoms of anxiety or clusters of symptoms, e.g. negative affect or psychological distress.

Similar to the studies of depressive symptoms and the menopausal transition, those of anxiety symptoms or distress have reported inconsistent results. For the most part, these studies have not used standardized measures of anxiety or distress but have included individual anxiety symptoms (e.g. irritability, tension) often as part of symptom checklists frequently used in studies of menopause [16–18]. The symptoms vary from study to study and may reflect those symptoms characterizing panic disorder (e.g. suddenly feeling fearful, heart pounding), social phobia (e.g. fear of social or performance situations), or generalized anxiety (e.g. excessive and uncontrollable worry, irritability). It is also the case that depressive and anxious symptoms overlap (e.g. fatigue, sleep disturbance are symptoms of both clinical depression and generalized anxiety disorder). Indeed studies have grouped anxious and depressive symptoms (e.g. irritability, tearfulness, feelings of panic) to represent psychological distress or negative mood [18–20].

Numerous older studies assessed a variety of anxiety symptoms [16, 21]. However, the limitations of the methodology including definitions of menopausal status, measurement of symptoms, and univariate analyses preclude meaningful results. More recent studies show some differences in associations between anxiety symptoms and menopausal stage.

Participants in the Melbourne Women's Midlife Health Project (MWMHP) reported nervous tension, with 33% bothered by the symptom during premenopause, 30% during early perimenopause, 40% during late perimenopause and 33% in the first year postmenopause. There were no significant differences across the Menopausal Transition stages [22].

An analysis of survey data from more than 15,000 women in the first stage of the Study of Women's Health Across the Nation (SWAN) [23] indicated that feeling tense or nervous was reported by 45% of premenopausal, 55% of early and late perimenopausal, and 50% of postmenopausal women. Prevalence rates of irritability were similar. In a subset of this cohort, odds of frequent (≥6 days in past 2 weeks) irritability and nervousness each adjusted for multiple covariates in separate analyses were significantly higher among early perimenopausal (OR = 1.33, 1.54, respectively) compared to premenopausal women [18].

The Penn Ovarian Aging (POA) study followed women aged 35–47 years old over 9 years and found that 19% of women reported anxiety during the premenopause, 24% during the early transition, and 19 and 16%, respectively, during the late transition and after menopause. In multivariable analyses, there was a trend (p = 0.09) for a menopause status effect with the early transition having significantly greater odds of anxiety (OR = 1.45, 95% CI = 1.05–2.01) than premenopause. Although prevalences were considerably higher for irritability, ranging from 31%-36% across menopausal stages, the differences were not significant [24].

Some studies, such as the MWMHP, included measures of constructs referred to as negative affect or psychological distress [19, 25]. In the MWMHP, across 6 annual assessments of mood in 354 Australian middle-aged women, negative mood (a subscale of the Affectometer-2) decreased over time [25]. The menopausal transition did not have a direct effect on negative mood, although symptoms did. In the 1946 British Cohort study, investigators also found no effect of menopausal status on psychological distress [19].

Factors Associated with Psychiatric Morbidity

Although psychiatric morbidity, as noted above, encompasses multiple symptoms and disorders, individual studies typically focus on specific symptoms or disorders as outcomes. Therefore, we discuss the factors associated with the specific outcomes reported. Variation in results may be due to differences in measures used to assess various outcomes. For example, depressive and anxious symptoms may be measured by self-administered questionnaires specifically designed to assess different types of symptoms. Other questionnaires may be designed to assess an overall negative affect or mood. Further, semi- or fully structured research interviews are used to ascertain diagnoses of disorder. Risk factors for psychiatric morbidity are organized according to the following domains: Psychosocial Factors, Health-Related Factors, and Lifetime Experiences and Exposures.

Psychosocial Factors

Several key psychosocial factors including sociodemographic, life stressors, social relations, and personality traits are associated with depression and may play a larger part in the development of depression than hormones or neurotransmitters in the brain.

Sociodemographic Factors

Studies of midlife women indicate that those with a high school education or less, or financial strain, and those who are separated, widowed, or divorced and in some studies, single, have a higher risk for depressive and anxious symptoms [4, 18, 26–30]. The limited data on racial/ethnic associations with depression among midlife women show mixed results [4, 26, 30] which may in part be due to different study designs and variables measured. For example, Bromberger et al. [4, 5] found in both cross-sectional and longitudinal analyses in SWAN that in unadjusted models African-American and Hispanic women had higher rates of elevated depressive symptoms whereas Chinese and Japanese women had lower rates compared to White women. The latter finding is consistent with previous studies. However, when adjusted for sociodemographics, health, and stressful events, there were no longer significant differences in the odds of symptoms between Whites and other racial/ethnic groups. In contrast to this US study, results of a cross-sectional study comparing symptom prevalence among 1,743 women, aged 40–60 years, living in Japan and Australia, found that the Japanese had higher rates of depressive symptoms [31]. This difference in the prevalence of depressive symptoms in US Japanese and indigenous Japanese relative to white women was also observed for nervousness.

Life Stressors

Psychosocial stress refers to environmental demands that tax or exceed the resources of the individual [32]. Such stress can be short-term or acute (e.g. loss of a job), or ongoing (e.g. financial strain, caring for sick or elderly relative, separation from spouse/partner, health problems in a spouse or child, or intimate partner violence) [33]. Stressful events have been associated with depression, anxiety, and negative mood syndromes [34]. The biological mechanisms associated with severe depression and psychosocial stress may be similar as they both involve dysregulation of the hypothalamic-pituitary-adrenal (HPA) axis. Over the last 25 years, research shows a consistent relationship between life stress and negative mood symptoms, including depression [34–36], with severe events more strongly associated with depression than nonsevere events [34, 36].

Multiple cross-sectional and prospective studies have shown that a variety of stressful events are correlated with or are risk factors for depressive and anxious symptoms among midlife women [5–7, 18, 27, 36–38]. Furthermore, most studies have indicated that such events are more strongly correlated with these symptoms [9, 19, 25, 27, 36–38] or disorder [39] than is menopausal status or vasomotor symptoms.

Studies report inconsistent findings with respect to whether the number of stressful events varies during the menopausal transition and whether this may account for differences in rates of depression during the transition [36, 39]. Several studies have observed an increased number of negative events in women aged 39–44 years. Among perimenopausal women, Schmidt et al. [39] found that clinically depressed women had more negative stressful events in the preceding 6 months than had nondepressed women (mean = 4.9 vs. 2.6 events, respectively).

Specific events, such as the departure of children from home, often referred to as the 'empty nest' were once thought to induce depression in middle-aged women, but empirical data do not consistently support such hypotheses [39–41]. Schmidt and Colleagues found that depressed perimenopausal women did not have more loss events, (e.g. a death in the family, departure of the last child from home, or divorce) compared to their nondepressed counterparts [39]. Similarly, longitudinal analyses of the MWMHP data over 9 years showed that in the first year after the last child departed, there was a reduction in negative mood. However, this was true only for those women at baseline who were not worried about children leaving home [41]. The latter finding suggests that there is likely individual variation linked to earlier factors in response to the departure of children from home. In a study of depressive symptoms conducted in the Netherlands among 2,700 middle-aged women, death of a partner or child increased the odds of high depressive symptoms by 1.56 and 5.87%, respectively [7]. Loss of a child however, occurs in only a very small proportion of middle-aged women and the death of a parent, a more common loss, did not significantly increase the odds of high symptoms in this study.

A key question is whether middle-age or the menopausal transition itself makes women more vulnerable to the negative effects of stress than does premenopause or postmenopause. A recent longitudinal study reported that among women experiencing a stressful event those who were perimenopausal compared to those who were premenopausal had a 2.4 odds of incident elevated depressive symptoms (CES-D ≥16) [9]. In the MWMHS, 3 or more daily hassles, and moderate or high interpersonal stress were associated with negative mood. Further, although the menopausal transition and hormone levels had no direct effects on negative mood, the menopausal transition interacted with paid work, self-rated health, and daily hassles to amplify the negative effects of these factors on mood [25].

Although stressful events may provoke depressive episodes, the large majority of individuals who experience stressful events or situations (other than extreme life stressors) do not become significantly depressed [34, 42]. A range of individual and social factors may explain differences in response to stress.

Social Relations

Depression, anxiety, and negative mood are associated with inadequate social support among midlife women [18, 19, 25] and in some cases, the association is independent of other relevant factors such as stressful life events [18]. The most salient type of social support is emotional support. It is the case, however, that many studies are cross-sectional and the direction of associations is confounded because a reduced interest in socializing is frequently a symptom or consequence of depression. Longitudinal studies address some of the confounding and suggest that low support is a risk factor for subsequent depression. Dennerstein et al. [25] found that the magnitude of negative mood was related to negative feelings for the partner or lack of a partner. In the SWAN, over 5 years of annual assessments, low social support was significantly associated with high depressive symptoms adjusting for multiple confounders, including stressful events and negative attitudes toward aging and menopause [5]. A longitudinal study of 524 middle-aged women found that multiple types of support, including perceived overall support, family and friends support, and marital satisfaction were correlated with depressive symptom levels at baseline and three years later adjusting for baseline value of social support [43]. This suggests that prior low social support may be a risk factor for subsequent depressive symptoms in midlife women.

Women provide and receive more support from other people and have more close friends than do men [42] suggesting that women would be protected more from depression than men. However, having a large social network is associated with increased risk for stressful events that occur to those with whom one is close [42]. Therefore, women are more likely than men to have interpersonal difficulties and conflicts which can contribute to depression [42] and negative mood [25].

Personality Traits

Personality traits or predispositions represent cognitive, affective, or behavioral tendencies that are relatively stable across time and situations. The classic female gender role is associated with traits of low instrumentality and high expressiveness. In a meta-analyses of 32 studies, Whitely [45] concluded that instrumentality (task or action oriented) was inversely associated with levels of depressive symptoms irrespective of gender. Similar results were reported in a recent longitudinal study of middle-aged women that statistically controlled for potential confounding [46]. In the Healthy Women Study (HWS), instrumentality, expressiveness, and depressive symptoms were measured at baseline with standard measures [46]. Three years later the less instrumental women showed a greater increase in depressive symptoms. Importantly, being highly expressive or nurturing was not associated with increased symptoms. Instrumentality is associated with active, problem-focused coping in stressful circumstances, which predicts psychological health in men and women [47]. The absence of this characteristic renders women particularly susceptible to depressive symptoms when stressed.

Other traits, including neuroticism or trait anxiety, pessimism, rumination and anger suppression have been associated with depressive symptoms and negative mood in studies of midlife women [19, 38, 46, 48]. Attitudes toward menopause and aging are conceptually related to pessimism and neuroticism and have been found to predict depressive and anxious symptoms and negative mood [5, 25, 28]. For example, in SWAN negative attitudes assessed at baseline nearly tripled the odds of a CES-D ≥16 over the next 5 years [5].

Personality traits may also render women susceptible to depression when they are exposed to stressful events as noted above or to changes in reproductive functioning. A propensity toward focusing on one's feelings when challenged or stressed has been correlated with negative affect [49]. In the HWS, middle-aged women who tended to hold anger in and subsequently initiated use of hormones had significantly higher mean Beck Depression symptom scores (mean = 5.4) than women who were low in anger suppression irrespective of menopausal status. In a study of midlife Danish women, those at the age of 40 who had high neuroticism were more likely to become hormone users at 45 years, but these results became nonsignificant when adjusted for potential confounders [50].

In the HWS, personality traits also interacted with chronic life stressors such that women who were highly internally focused at baseline and reported chronic problems three years later reported higher mean Beck Depression symptom scores (m = 6.3) than their counterparts who were less internally focused but also experienced chronic problems (mean = 4.2) [46]. A similar effect for the interaction between pessimism and chronic problems on high depressive symptoms was observed [38].

Health Behaviors, Physical Symptoms, and Conditions

Depression and anxiety are associated with high-risk health behaviors (During Midlife), including smoking, poor diet, inactivity, disturbed sleep [18, 24–26, 29, 51, 52] and lack of adherence to medical regimens. Depression and anxiety frequently coexist with medical illnesses including arthritis [18, 53], diabetes [54, 55], and cardiovascular conditions [56–58] and their risk factors. Further, the prevalence of depressive symptoms and disorder in medically ill patients is high, with estimates ranging from 15 to 53% depending on measures of depression and study design [59]. Physical illness can lead to depression and there is good evidence that depression itself is a risk factor for major conditions, such as diabetes [55].

Data regarding the relationship of body mass index to depressive symptoms and disorder have been inconsistent with some, but not all studies reporting significant positive associations between overweight and depression in midlife women [6, 8, 26, 60]. Roberts et al. [60] reported that 2,123 adults, aged 50 years and older, who were obese at baseline were twice as likely to be depressed 5 years later compared with those who were not obese.

In the Seattle Midlife Women's Health Study patterns of depressive symptom reporting annually over 6 years by 205 perimenopausal and postmenopausal women were evaluated. Results showed that a pattern of consistently high CES-D scores was associated with self-reported poor health in 1997, the start of the 6-year data collections [37]. Data from SWAN indicated that factors assessed at study entry, including poor/fair perceived health, high body pain and low role functioning predicted major or minor depression over the first 7 years of follow-up [unpubl. data].

Importantly, studies have documented significant associations between depressive and anxious symptoms and a variety of physical symptoms in midlife women [5, 15, 29]. For example, depressive symptoms have been correlated with dizzy spells, aches and stiff joints, diarrhea, and urinary incontinence [61]. Urinary incontinence has been associated with clinical depression [62].

Vasomotor Symptoms

Hot flashes and night sweats are the most prevalent symptoms during the menopausal transition and early postmenopause and are consistently associated with negative mood symptoms [5, 15, 18]. Most importantly, mood symptoms may affect quality of life among women with vasomotor symptoms. Considering the results of multiple studies of the menopausal transition, anxiety figures prominently in the experience of vasomotor symptoms during this period, although it is often analyzed as one of multiple symptoms in a cluster labeled 'negative affect' or 'psychological symptoms'. For example, in analyses of who was most bothered by hot flashes among the SWAN cohort, Thurston et al. [63] found that women with more negative affect, greater symptom sensitivity, more sleep problems and more frequent hot flashes and longer history of hot flashes found them most bothersome. Because the investigators included anxiety, as measured by the Spielberger State-Trait Anxiety Scale (trait) in a scale that also included measures of positive and negative affect, depressive symptoms, perceived stress, it is difficult to differentiate the influence of specific mood symptoms from negative affect or psychological distress.

The associations between negative mood symptoms and physical symptoms, including hot flashes and pain, for example, are bidirectional. That is, negative affect can influence perception and reporting of physical symptoms and as noted above, the latter can lead to depressed and anxious symptoms and disorder. The longitudinal studies of menopause and some preclinical studies suggest that anxious and depressive symptoms may induce disturbing or frequent vasomotor symptoms in some women [15, 29]. In SWAN, high scores on baseline anxiety and depressive symptom scores significantly increased the adjusted odds of frequent vasomotor symptoms (OR for anxiety = 3.10; OR for depressive symptoms = 1.62) over the subsequent 5 years [29]. Longitudinal data from the POA Study also found that the most anxious women had the most severe and most frequent vasomotor symptoms [15]. Anxiety at baseline predicted hot flashes 8–12 months later and there was a gradient of effect such that the most anxious women had the most frequent and severe symptoms. The relationship between hot flashes and anxiety persisted after adjusting for menopausal transition stage, depressed mood symptoms, smoking, BMI, estradiol, age, race, and time since the baseline measures in the study.

A recent review of studies of hot flashes and panic disorder points out many similarities between hot flashes and panic attacks [64]. The authors also suggest several models by which anxiety may affect hot flash experiences including the characteristics of anxious women that may make them more vulnerable to hot flashes. For example, anxiety sensitivity is a fear of arousal situations and it may be related to exaggerated symptom sensitivity. Such sensitivity could explain why subjective experiences of symptoms are in excess of objective recordings of symptoms as seen in Carpenter's studies of the objective and subjective experiences of hot flashes [65]. On the other hand, exaggerated autonomic nervous system responses associated with hot flashes may induce anxiety or feelings of loss of control. See Hanisch et al. [64] as this topic is outside the scope of this chapter.

Lifetime Experiences and Exposures

Numerous types of lifetime experiences contribute to the subsequent development of depression and anxiety. These include psychiatric history, reproductive characteristics and related psychiatric disorder/syndromes, childhood environment and adversity, and physical health history.

Psychiatric History

The best predictor of depressive and anxious symptoms and disorders in midlife is a past history of these disorders [24]. A recent prospective study of 266 middle-aged premenopausal and early perimenopausal women found that a history of an anxiety disorder was a significant predictor of incident major depression over 7 years, independent of vasomotor symptoms, stressful events, and role functioning [10]. In the POA, history of depression nearly doubled the odds of moderate or severe anxiety adjusted for multiple covariates including PMS history, perceived stress and hormone levels [24].

Studies of varying lengths have shown that psychological disorders in childhood and adolescence are significantly associated with mood and anxiety disorders in adulthood [66]. For example, data from the 1958 British Birth Cohort showed that childhood and adolescent externalizing and internalizing disorders Increased the odds of a depressive or anxiety disorder by 40–93% in men and women aged 45 years [66]. Thus, for some women, psychiatric disorders begin early in life. It is also the case that depressive syndromes or clinical episodes during midlife are associated with more recent periods of depression [67]. In the1946 British Birth Cohort, psychiatric illness lasting more than 1 year between ages 15 and 32 and 4 or more anxious and depressive symptoms at age 36 were significantly related to psychological symptoms when the women were 47–53 years old [19].

Health History

Most studies reporting a high prevalence of depression among the medically ill are cross-sectional. Such studies do not address the temporal relationship between the two. A few prospective studies of older adults indicate that physical illness can double the risk for the subsequent development of depression [59]. Thus, it is reasonable to consider prior health status as a risk factor for depression and possibly anxiety or negative mood during midlife and the menopausal transition. The few studies that have evaluated prior health showed equivocal results which may in part be due to the retrospective and crude nature of the self-reported medical history in these. In SWAN, women who had previously been told that they had anemia or migraines had significantly higher prevalences of CES-D scores ≥16 compared to their counterparts with scores <16, 29.1 vs. 21.4% for anemia and 33 vs. 22.4% for migraines [4]. However, only anemia remained a significant correlate of high CES-D in the multivariable analysis. This is unsurprising given that a cardinal symptom of depression is fatigue or lack of energy. Other conditions were not related to current CES-D. These analyses are limited by the retrospective self-report of medical history.

The longitudinal study of the 1946 British birth cohort collected information on childhood and adolescent characteristics and health problems and physical disability when women were 36 and 43 and assessed psychological symptom scores annually at ages 47–53 years. In multivariable analyses adjusting for multiple confounders including recent life stress and numbers of physical health problems, physical disability in prior adulthood was significantly positively associated with high psychological symptoms scores [19].

Reproductive Related Factors

Because mood and anxiety disorders are twice as prevalent among women as men, considerable attention has been given to the role of gonadal hormones in such disorders. Specific nuclear receptors for estrogens are found in many areas of the brain including the hippocampus, the hypothalamus and the medial amygdala. Steroid hormones can influence many aspects of neurotransmitter activity including the serotonin and norepinephrine systems that have been implicated in the development of depression [68]. It has been suggested that some women may be particularly vulnerable to mood disturbances during periods of hormonal variability within and across menstrual cycles which could modulate neurotransmitter systems in the brain [69].

Numerous studies of midlife women have reported associations between past premenstrual dysphoric disorder (PMDD) or premenstrual syndrome, typically referred to as PMS and of a lesser severity than PMDD, and anxiety and depression [26, 70, 71]. The MWMHS reported that among 290 women traversing the menopausal transition, past premenstrual physical and psychological complaints were significantly associated with high numbers of dysphoric symptoms over 3 years [71]. The POA found that a retrospective assessment of PMS at study entry doubled the odds of high depressive symptoms (CES-D $\geq$16) over 5 years [70] and was a consistent predictor of irritability, mood swings, anxiety and difficulty concentrating over the subsequent 9 years [24]. A limitation of this study is that only 22 of the 299 women providing data at the final end point were in the late stage of the menopausal transition and only 35 had become postmenopausal.

Other menstrual cycle characteristics may also be related to depression. For example, Harlow et al. [72] have shown that among women aged 36–45 who reported a younger age at menarche, and during the first 5 years of menstruation, number of days of flow ($\leq$3 and $\geq$7) compared to 4–6 days and moderate-heavy flow were associated with increased odds of subsequent major depression.

Childhood Abuse

Sexual abuse of children is much more common than was previously thought. Prevalence rates of childhood sexual abuse of girls in surveys of large nonclinical populations of adults in nearly two dozen countries have ranged from 7 to 36% [76]. Childhood sexual and physical abuse are associated with extensive mental health sequelae. For example, there is a substantial evidence showing long-term effects of childhood and adolescent abuse on the development and persistence of depression in adulthood [73–75]. Several mechanisms have been postulated to explain the effect of early sexual abuse in depression, including psychosocial factors such as guilt, low self-esteem, anxiety, helplessness [76] and neurobiological and neuroendocrine factors, such as HPA axis dysregulation [73, 77]. In SWAN, a history of early childhood abuse increased the risks of elevated depressive symptoms and major depression by twofold [78]. In the Seattle Midlife Women's Health Study, among 302 women followed for eight years, history of sexual abuse specifically was not significantly related to high depressive symptoms in multivariable analyses [6]. However, in this study only one question was used to assess sexual abuse history.

Both depressive and anxiety disorders are familial [79, 80]. Family studies show that women with major depression have more than a two fold risk of having a family member with depression than do those from the general population without depression [81]. Similar findings have been reported for the anxiety disorders with odds ratios ranging from 4.0 to 6.0 across all disorders for relatives of patients with an anxiety disorder. Panic disorder shows the strongest evidence for familial aggregation. Whether such findings are due to environmental or genetic influences has been examined in twin studies. The major source of familial risk for both major depression and anxiety disorders is genetic [80, 81].

Multiple genes and polymorphisms have shown potential associations with depression. No studies have assessed genetics for these disorders during the menopausal transition and only one has assessed genetics for depressive symptoms. The SWAN data showed that selected estrogen-related single nucleotide polymorphisms (SNPs) from 3 genes were associated with the CES-D score ≥ 16 in women who were premenopausal or perimenopausal and that the associations varied by ethnicity [82]. There are few studies of genetic polymorphisms that specifically account for anxiety disorders in midlife women. Nonetheless, there is growing understanding of the importance of genetic factors and anxiety in general [83]. Melke et al. [83] tested women born in 1956 (n = 251) for several types of anxiety finding that those who were homozygous for the short allele of the 5HTTLPR had higher anxiety scores than those who were heterozygous or who had two long alleles. Those with an intron 2 polymorphism had higher somatic anxiety symptoms.

Conclusion

Recent studies suggest that the menopausal transition is associated with negative mood and anxiety symptoms and syndromes and possibly clinical depression. Nevertheless, studies have also shown that multiple and varied psychosocial and health-related factors and lifetime exposures are related to negative mood and anxiety during the transition from the late reproductive years to postmenopause, often more strongly than is the stage of the transition. Many of these factors are not unique to midlife, but may converge with the biological and developmental changes of the menopausal transition to contribute to a constellation of mood and anxiety symptoms. Despite the large literature focused on the emotional concomitants of the menopausal transition and early postmenopause, the extent to which the transition may interact with the many factors discussed in this chapter to increase the risk for psychiatric morbidity remains unknown.

References

1 American Psychiatric Association: Diagnostic and Statistical Manual of Mental Disorders, ed 4. Washington, 1994.

2 Kessler RC, McGonagle KA, Swartz M, Blazer DG, Nelson CB: Sex and depression in the National Comorbidity Survey. I. Lifetime prevalence, chronicity and recurrence. J Affect Disord 1993;29:85–96.

3 Weissman MM, Bland R, Joyce PR, Newman S, Wells JE, Wittchen HU: Sex differences in rates of depression: cross-national perspectives. J Affect Disord 1993;29:77–84.

4 Bromberger JT, Harlow S, Avis N, Kravitz HM, Cordal A: Racial/ethnic differences in the prevalence of depressive symptoms among middle-aged women: the Study of Women's Health Across the Nation (SWAN). Am J Public Health 2004;94:1378–1385.

5 Bromberger JT, Matthews KA, Schott LL: Depressive symptoms during the menopausal transition: the Study of Women's Health Across the Nation (SWAN). J Affect Disord 2007;103:267–272.

6 Woods NF, Smith-Dijulio K, Percival DB, Tao EY, Mariella A, Mitchell S: Depressed mood during the menopausal transition and early postmenopause: observations from the Seattle Midlife Women's Health Study. Menopause 2008;15:223–232.

7 Maartens LW, Knottnerus JA, Pop VJ: Menopausal transition and increased depressive symptomatology: a community based prospective study. Maturitas 2002;42:195–200.

8 Freeman EW, Sammel MD, Lin H, Nelson DB: Associations of hormones and menopausal status with depressed mood in women with no history of depression. Arch Gen Psychiatry 2006;63:375–382.

9 Cohen LS, Soares CN, Vitonis AF, Otto MW, Harlow BL: Risk for new onset of depression during the menopausal transition: the Harvard study of moods and cycles. Arch Gen Psychiatry 2006;63:385–390.

10 Bromberger JT, Kravitz HM, Matthews K, Youlk A, Brown C, Feng W: Predictors of first lifetime episodes of major depression in midlife women. Psychol Med 2008:1–10.

11 Altemus M, Arleo EK: Gender differences in mood and anxiety disorders; in Leibenluft E (ed): Review of Psychiatry Series. Washington, American Psychiatric Press, 1999, pp 53–90.

12 Kessler RC, Berglund P, Demler O, Jin R, Merikangas KR, Walters EE: Lifetime prevalence and age-of-onset distributions of DSM-IV disorders in the National Comorbidity Survey Replication. Arch Gen Psychiatry 2005;62:593–602.

13 Halbreich U: Anxiety Disorders in Women: A developmental and lifecycle perspective. Depress Anxiety 2003;17:107–110.

14 Kessler RC: Epidemiology of women and depression. J Affect Disord 2003;74:5–13.

15 Freeman EW, Sammel MD, Lin H, Gracia CR, Kapoor S, Ferdousi T: The role of anxiety and hormonal changes in menopausal hot flashes. Menopause 2005;12:258–266.

16 Kaufert P, Syrotuik J: Symptom reporting at the menopause. Soc Sci Med [E] 1981;15:173–184.

17 Freeman EW, Sammel MD, Liu L, Martin P: Psychometric properties of a menopausal symptom list. Menopause 2003;10:258–265.

18 Bromberger JT, Assmann SF, Avis NE, Schocken M, Kravitz HM, Cordal A: Persistent mood symptoms in a multiethnic community cohort of pre- and perimenopausal women. Am J Epidemiol 2003;158:347–356.

19 Kuh D, Hardy R, Rodgers B, Wadsworth ME: Lifetime risk factors for women's psychological distress in midlife. Soc Sci Med 2002;55:1957–1973.

20 Bromberger JT, Meyer PM, Kravitz HM: Psychologic distress and natural menopause: a multiethnic community study. Am J Public Health 2001;91:1435–1442.

21 Jaszmann L, Van Lith ND, Zaat JC: The perimenopausal symptoms: the statistical analysis of a survey. Int J Fertil 1969;14:106–117.

22 Dennerstein L, Dudley EC, Hopper JL, Guthrie JR, Burger HG: A prospective population-based study of menopausal symptoms. Obstet Gynecol 2008;111:127–136.

23 Avis NE, Brockwell S, Colvin A: A universal menopausal syndrome? Am J Med 2005 December 19;118(suppl 12B):37–46.

24 Freeman EW, Sammel MD, Lin H, Gracia CR, Kapoor S: Symptoms in the menopausal transition: hormone and behavioral correlates. Obstet Gynecol 2008;111:127–136.

25 Dennerstein L, Lehert P, Burger H, Dudley E: Mood and the menopausal transition. J Nerv Ment Dis 1999;187:685–691.

26 Harlow BL, Cohen LS, Otto MW, Spiegelman D, Cramer DW: Prevalence and predictors of depressive symptoms in older premenopausal women: the Harvard Study of Moods and Cycles. Arch Gen Psychiatry 1999;56:418–424.

27 McKinlay JB, McKinlay SM, Brambilla D: The relative contributions of endocrine changes and social circumstances to depression in mid-aged women. J Health Soc Behav 1987;28:345–363.

28 Glazer G, Zeller R, Delumba L: The Ohio Midlife Women's Study. Health Care Women Int 2002;23: 612–630.

29 Gold EB, Sternfeld B, Kelsey JL: Relation of demographic and lifestyle factors to symptoms in a multiracial/ethnic population of women 40–55 years of age. Am J Epidemiol 2000;152:463–473.

30 Freeman EW, Sammel MD, Lin H: Symptoms associated with menopausal transition and reproductive hormones in midlife women. Obstet Gynecol 2007; 110(2 Pt 1):230–240.

31 Anderson D, Yoshizawa T, Gollschewski S, Atogami F, Courtney M: Menopause in Australia and Japan: effects of country of residence on menopausal status and menopausal symptoms. Climacteric 2004;7:165–174.

32 Lazarus R: Psychological Stress and Coping Process. New York, McGraw-Hill, 1966.

33 Caetano R, Cunradi C: Intimate partner violence and depression among Whites, Blacks, and Hispanics. Ann Epidemiol 2003;13:661–665.

34 Kessler RC: The effects of stressful life events on depression. Annu Rev Psychol 1997;48:191–214.

35 Brown GW, Bifulco A, Harris TO: Life events, vulnerability and onset of depression: some refinements. Br J Psychiatry 1987;150:30–42.

36 Greene JG, Cooke DJ: Life stress and symptoms at the climacterium. Br J Psychiatry 1980;136:486–491.

37 Woods NF, Mitchell ES: Pathways to depressed mood for midlife women: observations from the Seattle Midlife Women's Health Study. Res Nurs Health 1997;20:119–129.

38 Bromberger JT, Matthews KA: A longitudinal study of the effects of pessimism, trait anxiety, and life stress on depressive symptoms in middle-aged women. Psychol Aging 1996;11:207–213.

39 Schmidt PJ, Murphy JH, Haq N, Rubinow DR, Danaceau MA: Stressful life events, personal losses, and perimenopause-related depression. Arch Womens Ment Health 2004;7:19–26.

40 Radloff L: Depression and the empty nest. Sex Roles 1980;6:775–781.

41 Dennerstein L, Dudley E, Guthrie J: Empty nest or revolving door? A prospective study of women's quality of life in midlife during the phase of children leaving and re-entering the home. Psychol Med 2002;32:545–550.

42 Hammen C: Interpersonal stress and depression in women. J Affect Disord 2003;74:49–57.

43 Bromberger JT, Matthews KA: Employment status and depressive symptoms in middle-aged women: a longitudinal investigation. Am J Public Health 1994;84:202–206.

44 Fuhrer R, Stansfeld SA, Chemali J, Shipley MJ: Gender, social relations and mental health: prospective findings from an occupational cohort (Whitehall II study). Soc Sci Med 1999;48:77–87.

45 Whitely B: Sex-role orientation and psychological well-being: two meta-analyses. Sex Roles 1984;12: 207–225.

46 Bromberger JT, Matthews KA: A 'feminine' model of vulnerability to depressive symptoms: a longitudinal investigation of middle-aged women. J Pers Soc Psychol 1996;70:591–598.

47 Holohan C: Life stressors, personal and social resources, and depression: A 4-year structural model. J Abnorm Psychol 1991;100:131–138.

48 Lin MF, Ko HC, Wu JY, Chang FM: The impact of extroversion or menopause status on depressive symptoms among climacteric women in Taiwan: neuroticism as moderator or mediator? Menopause 2008;15:138–143.

49 Nolen-Hoeksema S, Morrow J, Fredrickson BL: Response styles and the duration of episodes of depressed mood. J Abnorm Psychol 1993;102:20–28.

50 Loekkegaard E, Epolv LF, Koster A, Garde K: Description of women's personality traits and psychological vulnerability prior to choosing hormone replacement therapy. Arch Womens Ment Health 2002;5:23–31.

51 Kravitz HM, Zhao X, Bromberger JT: Sleep disturbance during the menopausal transition in a multiethnic community sample of women. Sleep 2008; 31:979–990.

52 Elavsky S, McAuley E: Physical activity and mental health outcomes during menopause: a randomized controlled trial. Ann Behav Med 2007;33:132–142.

53 Wells KB, Rogers W, Burnam A, Greenfield S, Ware JE Jr: How the medical comorbidity of depressed patients differs across health care settings: results from the Medical Outcomes Study. Am J Psychiatry 1991;148:1688–1696.

54 Musselman DL, Betan E, Larsen H, Phillips LS: Relationship of depression to diabetes types 1 and 2: epidemiology, biology, and treatment. Biol Psychiatry 2003;54:317–329.

55 Everson-Rose SA, Meyer PM, Powell LH: Depressive symptoms, insulin resistance, and risk of diabetes in women at midlife. Diabetes Care 2004;27:2856–2862.

56 Glassman AH, Shapiro PA: Depression and the course of coronary artery disease. Am J Psychiatry 1998;155:4–11.

57 Jones DJ, Bromberger JT, Sutton-Tyrrell K, Matthews KA: Lifetime history of depression and carotid atherosclerosis in middle-aged women. Arch Gen Psychiatry 2003;60:153–160.

58 Agatisa PK, Matthews KA, Bromberger JT, Edmundowicz D, Chang YF, Sutton-Tyrrell K: Coronary and aortic calcification in women with a history of major depression. Arch Intern Med 2005; 165:1229–1236.

59 Creed F, Dickens C: Depression in the medically ill; in Steptoe A (ed): Depression and Physical Illness. New York, Camrbidge University Press, 2006, pp 3–18.

60 Roberts RE, Deleger S, Strawbridge WJ, Kaplan GA: Prospective association between obesity and depression: evidence from the Alameda County Study. Int J Obes Relat Metab Disord 2003;27:514–521.

61 Waetjen LE, Liao S, Johnson WO: Factors associated with prevalent and incident urinary incontinence in a cohort of midlife women: a longitudinal analysis of data: study of women's health across the nation. Am J Epidemiol 2007;165:309–318.

62 Nygaard I, Turvey C, Burns TL, Crischilles E, Wallace R: Urinary incontinence and depression in middle-aged United States women. Obstet Gynecol 2003;101:149–156.

63 Thurston RC, Bromberger JT, Joffe H: Beyond frequency: who is most bothered by vasomotor symptoms? Menopause 2008;15:841–847.

64 Hanisch LJ, Hansoo L, Freeman EW, Sullivan GM, Coyne JC: Hot flashes and panic attacks: a comparison of symptomatology, neurobiology, treatment, and a role for cognition. Psychol Bull 2008;134:247–269.

65 Carpenter JS, Azzouz F. Monahan PO, Storniolo AM, Rider SH: Is sterna skin conductance monitoring a Valis measure of hot flash intensity or distress? Menopause 2005;12:512–519.

66 Clark C, Rodgers B, Caldwell T, Power C, Stansfeld S: Childhood and adulthood psychological ill health as predictors of midlife affective and anxiety disorders: the 1958 British Birth Cohort. Arch Gen Psychiatry 2007;64:668–678.

67 Avis NE, Brambilla D, McKinlay SM, Vass K: A longitudinal analysis of the association between menopause and depression. Results from the Massachusetts Women's Health Study. Ann Epidemiol 1994;4:214–220.

68 McEwen BS, Alves SE: Estrogen actions in the central nervous system. Endocr Rev 1999;20:279–307.

69 Soares CN, Poitras JR, Prouty J: Effect of reproductive hormones and selective estrogen receptor modulators on mood during menopause. Drugs Aging 2003;20:85–100.

70 Freeman EW, Sammel MD, Rinaudo PJ, Sheng L: Premenstrual syndrome as a predictor of menopausal symptoms. Obstet Gynecol 2004;103(5 Pt 1): 960–966.

71 Morse C, Dudley E, Guthrie J, Dennerstein L: Relationships between premenstrual complaints and perimenopausal experiences. J Psychosom Obstet Gynecol 1998;19:182–191.

72 Harlow BL, Cohen LS, Otto MW, Spiegelman D, Cramer DW: Early life menstrual characteristics and pregnancy experiences among women with and without major depression: the Harvard study of moods and cycles. J Affect Disord 2004;79:167–176.

73 Weiss EL, Longhurst JG, Mazure CM: Childhood sexual abuse as a risk factor for depression in women: psychosocial and neurobiological correlates. Am J Psychiatry 1999;156:816–828.

74 Brown GW, Moran P: Clinical and psychosocial origins of chronic depressive episodes. I. A community survey. Br J Psychiatry 1994;165:447–456.

75 Riso LP, Miyatake RK, Thase ME: The search for determinants of chronic depression: a review of six factors. J Affect Disord 2002;70:103–115.

76 Trickett PK, Putnam F: Impact of child sexual abuse on females: toward a development psychological integration. Psychol Science 1993;4:81–87.

77 Penza KM, Heim C, Nemeroff CB: Neurobiological effects of childhood abuse: implications for the pathophysiology of depression and anxiety. Arch Womens Ment Health 2003;6:15–22.

78 Bromberger JT, Matthews KA, Goldbacher E, Brown C: Childhood abuse is associated with health and functioning in midlife African American and White women. Psychosom Med 2003;65:A72.

79 Bierut LJ, Health AC, Bucholz KK: Major depressive disorder in a community-based twin sample: are there different genetic and environmental contributions for men and women? Arch Gen Psychiatry 1999;56:557–563.

80 Hettema JM, Neale MC, Kendler KS: A review and meta-analysis of the genetic epidemiology of anxiety disorders. Am J Psychiatry 2001;158:1568–1578.

81 Sullivan PF, Neale MC, Kendler KS: Genetic epidemiology of major depression: review and meta-analysis. Am J Psychiatry 2000;157:1552–1562.

82 Kravitz HM, Janssen I, Lotrich FE, Kado DM, Bromberger JT: Sex steroid hormone gene polymorphisms and depressive symptoms in women at midlife. Am J Med 2006;119(9 suppl 1):S87–S93.

83 Melke J, Landen M, Baghei F: Serotonin transporter gene polymorphisms are associated with anxiety-related personality traits in women. Am J Med Genet 2001;105:458–463.

Joyce T. Bromberger, PhD
Associate Professor of Epidemiology and Psychiatry, University of Pittsburgh
3811 O'Hara Street
Pittsburgh, PA 15213 (USA)
Tel. +1 412 648 7108, Fax +1 412 648 7160, E-Mail brombergerjt@upmc.edu

Soares CN, Warren M (eds): The Menopausal Transition. Interface between Gynecology and Psychiatry.
Key Issues in Mental Health. Basel, Karger, 2009, vol 175, pp 66–76

Depression during the Perimenopausal Transition: What Have We Learned from Epidemiological Studies?

Sancia K. Ferguson · Claudio N. Soares · Bernard L. Harlow

Division of Epidemiology and Community Health, University of Minnesota, School of Public Health, Minneapolis, Minn., USA

Abstract

In this chapter, we provide a summary of the association between depression and the onset of the perimenopausal transition. We begin by summarizing the timing and classification criteria traditionally used to describe the perimenopausal transition. A discussion then follows regarding the accepted diagnostic criteria for determining new and recurrent onset of mood disorder, and difficult issues surrounding its measurement. We continue with a critical review of the literature on the association between depression and the perimenopausal transition, with particular attention being paid to issues of age at the time of the transition, the temporal relation between depression and the menopausal transition, and covariates that can influence the association. We conclude with a discussion of the importance of understanding the association and the need for further research to clarify the risks and benefits of hormone replacement therapy.   Copyright © 2009 S. Karger AG, Basel

The intent of this chapter is to systematically examine the findings from epidemiological studies on the association between depression and the perimenopausal transition. An explanation of how menopause and perimenopause are defined is a necessary foundation in unraveling what is known about this relationship. Equally relevant is how depression is defined both clinically and in the epidemiological literature. The definition of these terms can impact both the results of studies and the conclusions that are drawn. We discuss throughout this chapter the theory that perimenopause may constitute a vulnerable window due to hormonal fluctuations during which some women may be predisposed to depression, as well as a competing theory describing perimenopausal depression as a result of vasomotor symptoms, particularly sleep disturbances and nocturnal hot flashes. In addition, other covariates that may impact the relationship between perimenopause and depression are reviewed as well.

Epidemiology of Menoause and Perimenopause

The World Health Organization (WHO) defines natural menopause as the permanent cessation of menstruation resulting from the loss of ovarian follicular activity.
This is considered the gold standard in epidemiological literature, but must be determined retrospectively, following 12 consecutive months of amenorrhea without an
apparent underlying physiologic or pathologic cause [1, 2]. The average age of natural
menopause is estimated to be between the ages of 50 and 51 [1, 3, 4]. Age is often used
as a proxy for menopausal status. However, due to the wide variation in the actual
menopausal transition age, many premenopausal women are often misclassified as
menopausal, and vice versa [5, 6].

Perimenopause is defined by the World Health Organization as the aggregate of
the period of time immediately preceding final menses and the first year after menopause [1]. In the United States, the median age of onset for perimenopause is 47.5
years, with a range of persistence between 2 and 8 years, and an average duration of
4 years [5, 7]. Clinically, perimenopause is defined as the onset of menstrual irregularity, including shortened cycles or lengthened intervals of amenorrhea, as a consequence of the aging ovaries decreasing ability to respond to hormones [8]. As a result,
follicle-stimulating hormone (FSH) increases in an attempt to encourage the ovary
to respond [9]. Researchers have used FSH levels greater than 10–20 IU/l, or FSH
>25 IU/l as markers for perimenopause [10]. Other definitions employed to measure
perimenopause include self-reported variation in menstrual cycle length during the
previous 12 months [11–13], no menstrual cycles for 3–11 months [14, 15] and the
combination of cycle length changes of greater than 7 days' duration that occurred
with and without changes in menstrual flow amount, duration, or periods of amenorrhea for 3 months or longer [16, 17].

The perimenopause has also been further subdivided into early and late stages.
Early perimenopause has been defined as irregular bleeding in the previous 3 months
or change in cycle length over previous two cycles, while late perimenopause is
described as amenorrhea for 3–11 months [18] or alternatively as the 12 months preceding a consecutive period of amenorrhea for 3 months [19].

In 2001, a group of clinicians and researchers with expertise in reproductive aging
convened at the Stages of Reproductive Aging Workshop (STRAW) sponsored by
the American Society for Reproductive Medicine (ASRM), the National Institute
on Aging (NIA), the National Institute of Child Health and Human Development
(NICHD) and the North American Menopause Society. The goal was to (a) establish
a novel staging system for reproductive aging, (b) revise the perimenopausal nomen-
clature, and (c) identify areas for needed future research [20]. Using final menstrual
period (FMP) as time zero, the group identified seven unique stages of reproductive
aging as well as accompanying terminology. The 'reproductive' interval encompasses
stages –5 (early), –4 (peak), and –3 (late); the 'menopausal transition' interval includes
stages –2 (early) and stage –1 (late); and the 'postmenopause' interval includes stages

+1 (early) and +2 (late). According to the Straw criteria early perimenopause (–2) is characterized by variable cycle length greater than 2 days different from normal, and late perimenopause (–1) is characterized as more than 2 skipped cycles with accompanying amenorrhea. However, the committee also acknowledges that all women will not progress through each of the stages consecutively. There has been some criticism regarding whether the inclusion of hormonal levels such as FSH is premature, considering the variability among women, including young women with no fertility problems [21].

It has been suggested that race and ethnicity may have a role in the timing of menopause. However, this relationship has yet to be fully elucidated. Study design may contribute to the conflicting findings regarding differences in age at menopause among different races and ethnicities. A study by Harlow et al. [22] found that women of different ethnicities attribute different meaning to changes in their menstrual cycle. This underscores the need for a consistent and objective definition of menopause when making comparisons.

Over the last few decades, new instruments/tools have been developed to better characterize the clinical components of the menopausal transition and postmenopausal years. The Greene Climacteric Scale (GCS) was recently developed from a factor analysis of 30 symptoms reported by women 40–55 years of age. They were then grouped according to psychological, somatic and vasomotor symptoms [23]. Several studies found similar but not identical items to Greene's original 30 symptoms [24]. The 21-item scale was developed retaining 16 items from previous studies and using an additional four from later studies, with the addition of loss of sexual interest [23]. A four-point ranking scale is used to assess the presence, absence and severity of each of the 21 symptoms. The scale is unique because it does not attempt to composite a total score, but recognizes that symptoms arise from different domains, and provides a score for each of these. Another distinct aspect to this scale is the use of the psychological factor encompassing both anxiety and depression, which should be considered when comparing to studies using scales that specifically target depression.

Like the GCS, the Menopause Specific Quality of Life (MENQOL) takes a multifactorial approach to examining menopausal symptoms, but it differs in that it is designed to measure quality of life and responsiveness to change. A primary goal in developing the MENQOL was to create an instrument that would not only incorporate clinical elements, but would include the qualitative and quantitative aspects of a woman's individual experience, while simultaneously incorporating a scale of established psychometric properties. The investigators compiled a set of symptoms/problems commonly experienced by postmenopausal women, and conducted interviews to ensure its comprehensiveness. Participants were then asked if they had experienced the symptom in the past month, and, if so, rank its severity. The more disruptive the symptom and the more women experienced the symptom, the higher the composite score. The questions were assigned to specific domains including physical, psychosocial, vasomotor, and sexual. The scale was evaluated for reliability, validity, and responsiveness to change, and its ability to detect responsiveness to change makes it a good fit for studies evaluating interventions [25].

Epidemiology of Depression

Prior to the onset of puberty, the rates of depression in boys and girls are quite similar, with boys exhibiting a slight increase in prevalence over girls. However, following puberty this trend is altered. Women are more likely to experience major depressive disorder after puberty, with one population study demonstrating a 23% lifetime prevalence in women in comparison to 12.7% in men [26]. This phenomenon has been consistently observed throughout the world, although the magnitude of the female/male ratio fluctuates [27, 28]. It is not understood if this variance is real or due to inconsistency in how depression is defined or diagnosed [27].

According to the American Psychiatric Association, depression is characterized by a persistent downcast mood or loss of interest or pleasure (anhedonia). In addition, other symptoms often present include fatigue, unintentional weight loss, insomnia or hypersomnia, psychomotor agitation/retardation, fatigue or loss of energy, feelings of worthlessness or innapropriate/excessive guilt, diminished ability to concentrate or indecision, recurrent thoughts of death or suicide. The Diagnostic and Statistical Manual of Mental Disorders (DSM-IV) defines major depressive disorder (MDD) as any five or more of the previous symptoms with at least one of the symptoms being depressed mood or anhedonia within 2 weeks [29]. Historically, the terms minor depression, subsyndromal depression, and dysthymia have been used to describe depressive conditions with symptoms insufficient in severity or duration to meet the criteria for MDD, yet these symptoms continue to impact the lives and normal functioning of those afflicted [30, 31]. The DSM-IV identifies minor depressive disorder as a proposed diagnostic criteria, citing the need for more empirical validation. This potential category would be defined as having two to four symptoms of depression lasting for at least 2 weeks, excluding those with a previous diagnosis of MDD. Some researchers and clinicians have proposed a continuum model for depression, including minor depressive disorder and MDD as different manifestations of the same disorder. The models used to define depression and the methods used to measure it can significantly alter and impact the way in which we understand depression and its role in the perimenopausal transition.

There are several scales used in epidemiologic studies to access the presence of a broad range of depressive disorders, each with advantages and disadvantages. A common instrument that measures depressive symptoms in population-based studies is the Center for Epidemiologic Studies – Depression (CES-D) questionnaire [32]. The inventory is a 20-question self-report scale designed to measure depressive symptoms in community settings. It has been validated in many different populations and is considered reliable [33]. A score of 16 or more indicates the presence of depressive symptoms. A weakness of this instrument is its susceptibility to the influence of chronic medical conditions on the somatic subscale, possibly leading to an increase in scores. While some studies have used a score of 16 to encompass all depressive disorders, others have applied a score of 24 as a cutoff in an attempt to more closely approximate DSM-IV criteria for MDD. This can pose a problem when comparing the results of studies using the CES-D to that of other inventories.

The Hamilton Rating Scale for Depression (HAM-D) originally emerged in the 1960s and was designed to assess the severity of depression in those with a previous diagnosis of MDD, and continues to be a well-used inventory in mood disorder research [34]. This observer-based scale details parameters for its use including the independent rating of two researchers, incorporation of input from nurses and family members, and direct patient interview. An advantage of this scale is that an experienced rater can evaluate patients based on different parts of the depression spectrum. Another advantage is the multidimensional nature of the HAM-D, permitting 2 patients with the same score to have different combinations of items, suggesting different clinical outcomes [35]. Unfortunately, the importance of this differentiation is often ignored. The scale is commonly used to identify depression and/or recovery in subjects, and the implementation instructions are often disregarded [36]. There are two versions of the scale, one with 17 items and one with 21 items. The additional four items reflect less commonly occurring symptoms and significant confusion regarding which versions or subversions of these scales are implemented. The selected score set for diagnosis has been called arbitrary and has not been consistently used within the literature. Although the scales offer an attractive option for those studying mood disorders, misuse causes difficulty when comparisons are made between studies.

Recognizing the weaknesses of the HAM-D, Montgomery and Asberg designed a new scale, the Montgomery Asperg Depression Rating Scale (MADRS) which has grown in use. In a retrospective study comparing the MADRS to the HAM-D, MADRS was found to be as sensitive if not superior to the HAM-D in comparing treatment with antidepressants to placebo [35]. The scales are also comparable in their ability to measure severity and their ability to detect change. One advantage of using MADRS includes its ease of use. Uncomplicated language and directions and the equally weighted 10-item scale enable inexpert raters to reliably compute a score.

Age-Related Risk Factors for Depression during Perimenopause

Although women are born with 1–2 million ovarian follicles, at the onset of menarche only 500,000 follicles remain, and during the mid-40s perhaps only a few thousand [37]. Ovarian follicles decrease via one of two mechanisms: ovulation or atresia. Ovulation is the rupture of the follicle and subsequent release of the oocyte by the ovary. Atresia, the most common fate of a follicle, is a constant apoptotic degeneration of follicles beginning in utero and [38] continuing through menopause [39]. This decline in viable ovarian follicles is an important factor in the eventual cessation of menstruation. The few follicles that remain in the late reproductive years are quite resistant to rescue from atresia by FSH and unresponsive to luteinizing hormone (LH). The hypothalamus signals the pituitary to increase secretion of LH and FSH, in an ineffective effort to stimulate follicle maturity and combat falling estradiol levels. When this occurs in women younger than 40, and is accompanied by both amenorrhea and diminished estrogen levels, it is considered premature ovarian failure (POF) [40]. The etiology of POF is multi-factorial and the accelerated atresia is the result of genetic, immunologic, enzymatic, iatrogenic, toxic environmental and idiopathic causes [40]. The incidence of POF in the United States is estimated to be between 0.3 and 0.9% [41].

A predominance of studies have demonstrated that the highest prevalence of major depression in women occurs between ages 35 and 45 [28, 42] and coincides with diminishing circulating estrogen levels. However, there has been no clear evidence for increased rates of depression following menopause when estrogen levels remain low, and also no increased risk of depression in women with POF [43]. For this reason, proposed relationships between estrogen, premature menopause and depression place depression occurring prior to the premature termination of menstrual cycles. Women with POF or other causes of premature menopause could be subject to a more precipitous or qualitatively different decline in estrogen, potentially predisposing them to higher rates of depression [44]. In one study, 14% of those with POF had a history of depression in comparison to 6% in women who became menopausal after age 46 [45].

Association between Depression and Perimenopause

The theory that the menopausal transition is associated with an increased risk of depression has been consistently reshaped and refined as we come to better understand the mechanisms of this process. Despite extensive study of perimenopause, the nature of its relationship to depression is still not fully understood and remains somewhat controversial. An evolving theory is a model of perimenopause as a 'window of vulnerability' in a woman's life. During perimenopause, women are thought to be at higher risk for developing depression due to fluctuations in hormone levels, independent of the absolute hormone levels [46]. Fluctuating hormone levels may have an impact on estrogen's ability to synthesize and augment the effects of the monoaminergic systems in the limbic system, hippocampus, and amygdala, areas of the brain that participate in emotional processing and mood regulation [47]. There is a growing body of evidence for perimenopause as a window of vulnerability for depression. Recent data from a cross-sectional study of 421 women in the Harvard Study of Moods and cycles demonstrates that perimenopausal women with no lifetime history of major depression were twice as likely (OR 1.9; 95% CI 0.9–4.0) to develop depression than premenopausal women after adjusting for both age at study enrollment and history of negative life events [48]. In an 8-year longitudinal study of 251 women, Freemen et al. [18] reported that women entering the perimenopausal transition were 2.5 times more likely to report a depression diagnosis compared to women remaining premenopausal (OR 2.5; 95% CI 1.25–5.0). Participants in the multiethnic multicentered Study of Women's Health Across the Nation (SWAN) reported increased depressive symptoms during perimenopause in comparison to premenopausal women (OR range 1.30–1.71) [49]. All three studies defined perimenopause similarly and used the CES-D for assessing depressive symptoms.

Further longitudinal studies of perimenopause and depression support these findings [11, 13, 50]. Additionally, Avis et al. [51] and Dennerstein et al. [19] report that women with longer duration of perimenopause have increased rates of depression compared to women with shorter duration of perimenopause. There is evidence that women who have had episodes of reproductive-related depression, including premenstrual symptoms, symptoms during pregnancy, postpartum, or when beginning or ending hormonal contraceptives, have an increased risk of recurrent depression during perimenopause [52–54]. Rather than an isolated window of vulnerability, these women are thought to have multiple windows of vulnerability or a continuum of increased risk [55].

Some researchers assert that depression during perimenopause is not the direct result of hormonal fluctuations, but rather a consequence of vasomotor symptoms, specifically the sleep disruptions caused by nocturnal hot flashes. While this trend is demonstrated in the literature, it does not tell the whole story. Joffe et al. [12] reported that women experiencing vasomotor symptoms during perimenopause were at four times greater risk of experiencing depression than their counterparts with no vasomotor symptoms, irrespective of a past history of depression. Findings from the Seattle Midlife Women's Health Study also demonstrated an association between sleep disruption, the presence of hot flashes, and higher depressive scores [56]. In support of a theory of hormonal fluctuations, depression has been observed during the menopausal transition without the presence of vasomotor symptoms or sleep disruption, and can be successfully treated by agents that do not target vasomotor symptoms [57]. Data from Cohen et al. [48] do, however, indicate an increased risk of depression for perimenopausal women experiencing vasomotor symptoms, compared to perimenopausal women without vasomotor symptoms and premenopausal women (OR 2.2, 95% CI 1.1 <4.2). The use of estrogen replacement as an effective antidepressant in perimenopausal women, but not postmenopausal women, also supports the theory that hormone fluctuation may be responsible for depression during perimenopause. Transdermal estradiol was found to successfully treat depression in two independent studies [50, 58]. Several studies examining the role of hormone replacement therapy (HRT) as a mechanism for treating depression fail to make a distinction between post menopausal and perimenopausal women in their study populations [59], making extrapolation of the results difficult. Current recommendations include the addition of estrogen/progesterone to selective serotonin reuptake inhibitors (SSRI) when treating refractory depression in perimenopausal or postmenopausal women [59].

Covariates that May Have an Impact on the Relationship between Depression and Menopausal Transition

Factors that impact age at menopausal onset include age at menarche, menstrual cycle length, hormonal contraceptive use, and parity. These factors determine the lifetime number of ovulatory cycles a woman experiences. Several studies have examined the individual contributions of each of these factors to early menopause. An earlier age at menarche may be related to earlier onset of menopause by shifting the reproductive period earlier. Although one study found that an early onset of menarche was associated with early menopause [37], other studies found no association [60–62]. In theory, women with shorter cycles, particularly during the early reproductive years, will ovulate more frequently than women with longer cycles, depleting viable follicles more rapidly, decreasing the age at menopause by 1–2 years [62]. Pregnancy and hormonal contraceptive use halt ovulation, increasing age of menopausal onset. Both an older age at menopause for multiparious women and a younger age at menopause for nulliparious women have been illustrated [3, 62–65]. The role of hormonal contraception remains unclear, with some studies indicating that use decreases age at menopause [61], while other studies observe no association [3, 63].

Cigarette smoking is consistently and strongly linked to a decreased age at menopause by about 1 year [3]. Nicotine and anabasine, alkaloid components of tobacco smoke, likely inhibit estrogen synthesis via inhibition of granulosa cell aromatase and other enzymes critical to estrogen production [66]. Additionally, polycyclic hydrocarbons found in tobacco smoke are thought to be harmful to ovarian germ cells, leading to estrogen deficiency and follicular exhaustion [67]. Less active estrogens may be observed in smokers due to favoring of 2-hydroxylation over 16-hydroxylation of estrogen [68]. At least one cross-sectional study identified an association between depressive symptoms and smoking among premenopausal women of late reproductive age [15]. The roles of cigarette smoking and depression in perimenopause have yet to fully be elucidated. They may act independently, influencing the onset of menopause and the severity of menopausal symptoms, or they may interact with each other to influence menopausal transition and somatic symptoms.

The role of body mass index and the timing of menopausal onset remain controversial. While one study found that overweight and obese women (BMI >25) experienced menopause about 1 year earlier than nonobese women, another found no association of BMI with age at menopausal onset [63]. Notably in this study, however, women trying to lose weight by diet restriction, or who gained 27 or more pounds experienced menopause about 1 year earlier than their counterparts.

Conclusion

Although the majority of women do not experience depression during perimenopause, it remains important to be aware of the increased risk of depression during this vulnerable time. The most recent studies not only suggest a relationship between perimenopause and depression, but indicate depression is more likely to occur in the later stages of perimenopause. A longer length of perimenopause as well as the accompaniment of vasomotor symptoms further increases this risk. As record numbers of women enter menopause, it is critical that clinicians are aware of this increased risk in order to promote the safety and well-being of their patients. To ensure the success of this endeavor, we must continue to explore appropriate therapeutic options, including the potential role of hormonal and nonhormonal interventions. As the risks and benefits of hormone replacement are examined, and the subsets of women who can use it safely are identified, we should also evaluate the efficacy of complimentary medical therapies, which are becoming increasingly prevalent.

References

1 World Health Organization Scientific Group: Research on the Menopause. WHO Technical Services Report Series, 1981, p 670.
2 Harlow BL, Signorello LB: Factors associated with early menopause. Maturitas 2000;35:3–9.
3 Bromberger JT, Matthews KA, Kuller LH, Wing RR, Meilahn EN, Plantinga P: Prospective study of the determinants of age at menopause. Am J Epidemiol 1997;145:124–133.
4 Cramer DW, Xu H: Predicting age at menopause. Maturitas 1996;23:319–326.
5 McKinlay SM, Brambilla DJ, Posner JG: The normal menopause transition. Maturitas 1992;14:103–115.
6 Morabia A, Costanza MC: International variability in ages at menarche, first livebirth, and menopause. world health organization collaborative study of neoplasia and steroid contraceptives. Am J Epidemiol 1998;148:1195–1205.
7 Treloar AE, Boynton RE, Behn BG, Brown BW: Variation of the human menstrual cycle through reproductive life. Int J Fertil 1967;12(1 Pt 2):77–126.
8 Speroff L: The perimenopausal transition. Ann NY Acad Sci 2000;900:375–392.
9 Fitzgerald CT, Seif MW, Killick SR, Elstein M: Age related changes in the female reproductive cycle. Br J Obstet Gynaecol 1994;101:229–233.
10 Rasgon N, Shelton S, Halbreich U: Perimenopausal mental disorders: Epidemiology and phenomenology. CNS Spectr 2005;10:471–478.
11 Bromberger JT, Assmann SF, Avis NE, Schocken M, Kravitz HM, Cordal A: Persistent mood symptoms in a multiethnic community cohort of pre- and perimenopausal women. Am J Epidemiol 2003;158:347–356.
12 Joffe H, Hall JE, Soares CN, Hennen J, Reilly CJ, Carlson K, et al: Vasomotor symptoms are associated with depression in perimenopausal women seeking primary care. Menopause 2002;9:392–398.
13 Maartens LW, Knottnerus JA, Pop VJ: Menopausal transition and increased depressive symptomatology: a community based prospective study. Maturitas 2002;42:195–200.
14 Owens JF, Matthews KA: Sleep disturbance in healthy middle-aged women. Maturitas 1998;30:41–50.
15 Hyde Riley E, Inui TS, Kleinman K, Connelly MT: Differential association of modifiable health behaviors with hot flashes in perimenopausal and postmenopausal women. J Gen Intern Med 2004;19:740–746.
16 Binfa L, Castelo-Branco C, Blumel JE, Cancelo MJ, Bonilla H, Munoz I, et al: Influence of psycho-social factors on climacteric symptoms. Maturitas. 2004;48:425–431.

17 Harlow BL, Wise LA, Otto MW, Soares CN, Cohen LS: Depression and its influence on reproductive endocrine and menstrual cycle markers associated with perimenopause: the Harvard study of moods and cycles. Arch Gen Psychiatry 2003;60:29–36.

18 Freeman EW, Sammel MD, Liu L, Gracia CR, Nelson DB, Hollander L: Hormones and menopausal status as predictors of depression in women in transition to menopause. Arch Gen Psychiatry 2004;61:62–70.

19 Dennerstein L, Guthrie JR, Clark M, Lehert P, Henderson VW: A population-based study of depressed mood in middle-aged, Australian-born women. Menopause 2004;11:563–568.

20 Soules MR, Sherman S, Parrott E, et al: Executive summary: Stages of reproductive aging workshop (STRAW). Fertil Steril 2001;76:874–878.

21 Den Tonkelaar I, Broekmans FJ, De Boer EJ, Te Velde ER, Soules MR, Parrott E, et al: The stages of reproductive aging workshop. Menopause. 2002; 9:463,4; author reply 464–465.

22 Harlow SD, Crawford SL, Sommer B, Greendale GA: Self-defined menopausal status in a multi-ethnic sample of midlife women. Maturitas 2000;36:93–112.

23 Greene JG: Constructing a standard climacteric scale. Maturitas 1998;29:25–31.

24 Hunter M, Battersby R, Whitehead M: Relationships between psychological symptoms, somatic complaints and menopausal status. Maturitas 1986;8:217–228.

25 Hilditch JR, Lewis J, Peter A, van Maris B, Ross A, Franssen E, et al: A menopause-specific quality of life questionnaire: development and psychometric properties. Maturitas 1996;24:161–175.

26 Kessler RC, McGonagle KA, Nelson CB, Hughes M, Swartz M, Blazer DG: Sex and depression in the national comorbidity survey. II. Cohort effects. J Affect Disord 1994;30:15–26.

27 Grigoriadis S, Robinson GE: Gender issues in depression. Ann Clin Psychiatry. 2007;19:247–255.

28 Weissman MM, Bland RC, Canino GJ, Faravelli C, Greenwald S, Hwu HG, et al: Cross-national epidemiology of major depression and bipolar disorder. JAMA 1996;276:293–299.

29 American Psychiatric Association: Diagnostic and Statistical Manual of Mental Disorders, ed 4. Washington, 1994.

30 Angst J, Merikangas KR, Preisig M: Subthreshold syndromes of depression and anxiety in the community. J Clin Psychiatry 1997;58(suppl 8):6–10.

31 Rapaport MH, Judd LL, Schettler PJ, et al: A descriptive analysis of minor depression. Am J Psychiatry 2002;159:637–643.

32 Radloff LS: The CES-D scale: A self-report depression scale for research in the general population. Appl Psychol Measurem 1977;1:385.

33 Knight RG, Williams S, McGee R, Olaman S: Psychometric properties of the centre for epidemiologic studies depression scale (CES-D) in a sample of women in middle life. Behav Res Ther 1997; 35:373–380.

34 Hamilton M: A rating scale for depression. J Neurol Neurosurg Psychiatry 1960;23:56–62.

35 Khan A, Leventhal RM, Khan SR, Brown WA: Severity of depression and response to antidepressants and placebo: an analysis of the food and drug administration database. J Clin Psychopharmacol 2002;22:40–45.

36 Snaith RP: Present use of the Hamilton depression rating scale: observation on method of assessment in research of depressive disorders. Br J Psychiatry 1996;168:594–597.

37 Cramer DW, Xu H, Harlow BL: Does 'incessant' ovulation increase risk for early menopause? Am J Obstet Gynecol 1995;172:568–573.

38 Hsueh AJ, Billig H, Tsafriri A: Ovarian follicle atresia: a hormonally controlled apoptotic process. Endocr Rev 1994;15:707–724.

39 Tilly JL, Kowalski KI, Johnson AL, Hsueh AJ: Involvement of apoptosis in ovarian follicular atresia and postovulatory regression. Endocrinology 1991;129:2799–2801.

40 de Moraes-Ruehsen M, Jones GS: Premature ovarian failure. Fertil Steril. 1967;18:440–461.

41 Coulam CB, Adamson SC, Annegers JF: Incidence of premature ovarian failure. Obstet Gynecol 1986; 67:604–606.

42 Blazer DG, Kessler RC, McGonagle KA, Swartz MS: The prevalence and distribution of major depression in a national community sample: The national comorbidity survey. Am J Psychiatry 1994;151:979–986.

43 de Taraciuk MB, Nolting M, Fernandez G, Colela D, Onetto C, Straminsky V: Psychological assessment of patients with premature ovarian failure. Gynecol Endocrinol 2008;24:44–53.

44 Harlow BL, Signorello LB: Factors associated with early menopause. Maturitas. 2000;35:3–9.

45 Harlow BL, Cramer DW, Annis KM: Association of medically treated depression and age at natural menopause. Am J Epidemiol 1995;141:1170–1176.

46 Rubinow DR, Schmidt PJ, Roca CA: Estrogen-serotonin interactions: implications for affective regulation. Biol Psychiatry 1998;44:839–850.

47 Stahl SM: Effects of estrogen on the central nervous system. J Clin Psychiatry 2001;62:317–318.

48 Cohen LS, Soares CN, Vitonis AF, Otto MW, Harlow BL: Risk for new onset of depression during the menopausal transition: the Harvard study of moods and cycles. Arch Gen Psychiatry 2006;63:385–390.

49 Bromberger JT, Matthews KA, Schott LL, Brockwell S, Avis NE, Kravitz HM, et al: Depressive symptoms during the menopausal transition: the Study of Women's Health Across the Nation (SWAN). J Affect Disord 2007;103:267–272.

50 Schmidt PJ, Haq N, Rubinow DR: A longitudinal evaluation of the relationship between reproductive status and mood in perimenopausal women. Am J Psychiatry 2004;161:2238–2244.

51 Avis NE, Brambilla D, McKinlay SM, Vass K: A longitudinal analysis of the association between menopause and depression: results from the massachusetts women's health study. Ann Epidemiol 1994;4:214–220.

52 Boyd RC, Amsterdam JD: Mood disorders in women from adolescence to late life: an overview. Clin Obstet Gynecol 2004;47:515–526.

53 Steiner M, Dunn E, Born L: Hormones and mood: from menarche to menopause and beyond. J Affect Disord 2003;74:67–83.

54 Stewart DE, Boydell KM: Psychologic distress during menopause: associations across the reproductive life cycle. Int J Psychiatry Med 1993;23:157–162.

55 Soares CN: Depression during the menopausal transition: window of vulnerability or continuum of risk? Menopause 2008;15:207–209.

56 Woods NF, Smith-DiJulio K, Percival DB, Tao EY, Mariella A, Mitchell S: Depressed mood during the menopausal transition and early postmenopause: observations from the Seattle Midlife Women's Health Study. Menopause 2008;15:223–232.

57 Soares CN, Joffe H, Rubens R, Caron J, Roth T, Cohen L: Eszopiclone in patients with insomnia during perimenopause and early postmenopause: a randomized controlled trial. Obstet Gynecol 2006; 108:1402–1410.

58 Soares CN, Almeida OP, Joffe H, Cohen LS: Efficacy of estradiol for the treatment of depressive disorders in perimenopausal women: a double-blind, randomized, placebo-controlled trial. Arch Gen Psychiatry 2001;58:529–534.

59 Parry BL: Perimenopausal depression. Am J Psychiatry 2008;165:23–27.

60 Parazzini F, Negri E, La Vecchia C: Reproductive and general lifestyle determinants of age at menopause. Maturitas 1992;15:141–149.

61 Stanford JL, Hartge P, Brinton LA, Hoover RN, Brookmeyer R: Factors influencing the age at natural menopause. J Chronic Dis 1987;40:995–1002.

62 Whelan EA, Sandler DP, McConnaughey DR, Weinberg CR: Menstrual and reproductive characteristics and age at natural menopause. Am J Epidemiol 1990;131:625–632.

63 Brambilla DJ, McKinlay SM: A prospective study of factors affecting age at menopause. J Clin Epidemiol 1989;42:1031–1039.

64 Jeune B: Parity and age at menopause in a Danish sample. Maturitas 1986;8:359–365.

65 Stanford JL, Hartge P, Brinton LA, Hoover RN, Brookmeyer R: Factors influencing the age at natural menopause. J Chron Dis 1987;40:995–1002.

66 Barbieri RL, McShane PM, Ryan KJ: Constituents of cigarette smoke inhibit human granulosa cell aromatase. Fertil Steril 1986;46:232–236.

67 Mattison DR, Thorgeirsson SS: Smoking and industrial pollution, and their effects on menopause and ovarian cancer. Lancet 1978;i:187–188.

68 Michnovicz JJ, Hershcopf RJ, Naganuma H, Bradlow HL, Fishman J: Increased 2-hydroxylation of estradiol as a possible mechanism for the anti-estrogenic effect of cigarette smoking. N Engl J Med 1986; 315:1305–1309.

Bernard L. Harlow, PhD
Division of Epidemiology, University of Minnesota
1300 S 2nd St, Room 300 WBOB
Minneapolis, MN 55454 (USA)
Tel. +1 612 626 6527, Fax +1 612 624 0315, E-Mail harlow@umn.edu

Soares CN, Warren M (eds): The Menopausal Transition. Interface between Gynecology and Psychiatry.
Key Issues in Mental Health. Basel, Karger, 2009, vol 175, pp 77–87

Thermoregulation and Menopause: Understanding the Basic Pathophysiology of Vasomotor Symptoms

Darlene C. Deecher

Women's Health, Wyeth Research, Collegeville, Pa., USA

Abstract

Women have sought treatment for vasomotor symptoms (VMS) associated with menopause for decades. Common terms that describe VMS are hot flashes/flushes and night sweats. Research in this field has yet to elucidate the biological details explaining the causes of VMS. The need to develop additional therapies that can treat VMS has shifted the focus of research from hormonal treatments (i.e. estrogens and progestins) to investigating the biological processes involved in hormone-dependent temperature regulation. The basic underlying premise is that VMS occur due to a disruption in pathways modulated by ovarian hormones that maintain temperature homeostasis. Disruption in this tightly controlled temperature circuit causes an exaggerated heat-loss response resulting in an intense feeling of heat followed by skin reddening and sequentially sweating. Changes in ovarian hormone levels during menopause impact multiple components involved in temperature maintenance. Understanding the pathways and mechanisms involved in temperature regulation and elucidating specific receptors or neurotransmitters implicated in thermoregulatory dysfunction will guide future understanding of VMS causality and drug discovery efforts. This chapter reviews what is currently known about temperature regulation, and the impact of fluctuating and declining ovarian hormone levels on this regulation that lead to temperature dysfunction resulting in VMS.

Copyright © 2009 S. Karger AG, Basel

Vasomotor symptoms (VMS) are considered the hallmark of the menopausal transition. The prevalence rate of these symptoms has been reported to be between 60 and 88% in women during this time period [1, 2]. Vasomotor symptoms encompass the symptoms that women commonly refer to as hot flashes/flushes and night sweats. Other terms that are often associated with VMS include vasomotor dysfunction, vasomotor disturbances, vasomotor instability, vasomotor disorders, thermoregulatory disorders or thermoregulatory dysfunction. While the causes of VMS are not precisely known, the symptoms are associated with changes in ovarian hormone levels and function. It is well established that hormone-containing therapies provide effective dose-related relief [3].

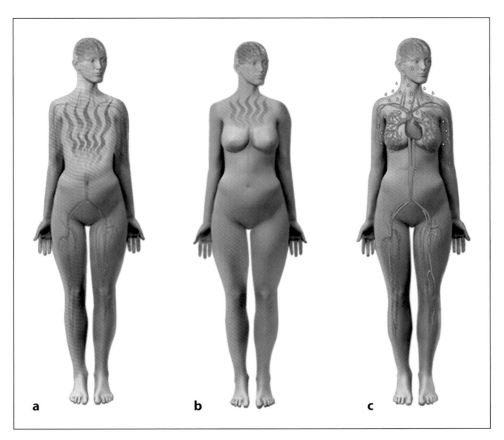

Fig. 1. Typical physical signs denoted by patients experiencing severe vasomotor symptoms. **a** Flash; sudden intense heat sensation. **b** Flush; skin reddening spreading from chest to face. **c** Sweat; blood vessels dilate, heat is dissipated via skin and sweat glands activated.

The common descriptors of VMS reported by women include 3 characteristics (fig. 1). Women may experience all or some of these signs during a hot flash event. Typically, the onset of a hot flash starts with a sudden and transient sensation of intense heat (flash; fig. 1a) that initiates the reddening in the upper torso that spreads over the chest and face (flush; fig. 1b) accompanied by sweating (fig. 1c). In some cases, women may experience the sensation of chills followed by shivering. Additionally women have reported experiencing palpitations or feelings of anxiety during a hot flash event. Night sweats are part of moderate-to-severe VMS and typically occur during sleep. They are described as drenching diaphoresis and cause sleep disturbances resulting in diminished sleep quality. In general, the majority of women reporting moderate to severe VMS will identify with these signs but not all women will necessarily recognize or experience all of these. In addition, the poor sleep quality reported by women experiencing VMS has been associated with fatigue, lethargy, inability to concentrate, lack of motivation, difficulty performing tasks, an increase in tension/irritability and dysphoria. Thus, taken together, moderate to severe VMS can have a negative impact on the quality of life and functional abilities of the individual experiencing these symptoms [1].

The occurrence of VMS varies in frequency from several times per week to more than 15 per day dependent on the individual woman and severity of the symptoms. They sometimes occur several times within 1 h and often occur at night, resulting in sleep disruptions. The Gothenburg longitudinal study took a closer look at the occurrence of VMS in the same group of women over a 25-year time period [1]. This study showed the peak incidence of VMS occurs between 52 and 54 years of age with symptoms beginning several years prior to menopause. Women reported VMS as early as 38 years of age. It should be noted that the earliest age in this study was 38, so it is possible that VMS can occur earlier. The mean duration of symptoms have been reported to be approximately 3 years; however, as many as 60% of women experience VMS for up to 7 years. Additionally, up to 15% of women experience VMS for more than 15 years after menopause. In summary, the findings from this study indicate that VMS may start prior to the onset of the menopause transition and can last well beyond menopause in some women. Thus, the majority of women going through menopause will experience these symptoms however the severity, frequency and duration are individualized. Currently, the science is lacking to explain or identify which individuals will be affected by VMS or the prediction of the severity and impact on daily life activities.

Although VMS are commonly reported by women who are transitioning through menopause or who are menopausal as a result of surgery, other populations report experiencing these symptoms. These populations include women approaching menopause (perimenopausal; perimenopause is part of the menopausal transition) as suggested by the findings of the Gothenburg study [1]. Typically, these women experience VMS in association with changes in the menstrual cycle (i.e. duration or frequency). These symptoms are often severe, but transient, with the frequency increasing as a woman approaches menopause. Also, women will experience VMS when taking medications that disrupt the balance of the hypothalamic-pituitary-gonadal axis. These types of drugs are gonadotropin-releasing hormone (GnRH) analogs, estrogen receptor antagonists in the brain [4] (i.e. raloxifene and tamoxifen) or aromatase inhibitors [5]. Vasomotor symptoms are not solely gender specific. They are reported by hypogonadal men and men experiencing age-associated androgen decline as well as by men undergoing androgen-ablation therapy (e.g. GnRH analogs) for prostate cancer [6]. Additionally, VMS are reported by men with an abrupt loss of testicular function after orchidectomy for the treatment of prostatic testicular cancer and following certain procedures that compromise testicular function. Thus, men have reported frequent and severe VMS that disrupt their daily activities. In summary, both women and men have reported experiencing moderate to severe VMS. These symptoms appear to be associated with gonadal hormone fluctuation or decline and are debilitating, disruptive and bothersome in these reported populations. It is safe to propose that changes in gonadal hormone levels are directly causal to VMS.

Additionally, it is well established that hormone-based therapies provide effective relief to patients with moderate to severe VMS associated with menopause. However, some populations who experience VMS are either contraindicated or unsuitable for prescribing hormone-containing therapies. Therefore, an unmet medical need exists for the development of a safe and effective nonhormonal treatment to complement existing approved therapies.

Temperature Regulation

It is thought that VMS are a result of a malfunction or disruption in communication within a complex temperature circuit that controls temperature regulation [3]. The goal of this regulation is to maintain a constant body temperature in order to allow for optimal organ function and maintenance of overall homeostatic processes. Maintaining consistent and precise internal body temperature (37°C) requires coordinated and succinct communication between three major control sites. These major coordinating centers are the brain, the internal body cavity and the skin (fig. 2). A complex communication network coordinates information between these major control sites in order to maintain constant internal body temperature independent of external temperature changes. The thermoregulatory circuitry is responsible for initiating heat dissipation/retention or generation of activities as needed in response to internal and external stimuli [7]. All of these activities are controlled and regulated by a group of temperature-sensitive neurons located in a region of the brain called the hypothalamus (fig. 2, top) that act as the body's thermostat [8]. The hypothalamus receives data from thermal receptors both inside and outside the central nervous system. As a result, it can sense changes in the internal body core (cranial, thoracic and abdominal) (fig. 2, middle) as well as the shell (skin, subcutaneous tissue and muscle) temperature (fig. 2, bottom) [7]. It then produces the necessary adjustments in internal body temperature via controlled release of hormones and neurotransmitters [9].

If core or skin temperatures increase, the hypothalamic neurons send signals that cause subcutaneous blood vessel dilation [7, 9]. Peripheral vasodilation results in an increase in blood volume and flow to the skin allowing heat loss by various processes including sweating and evaporation (fig. 2, bottom). The peripheral vasodilation process is a means of transferring heat from the internal body cavity (core) to the skin. Concurrently, the hypothalamus inhibits the release of hormones that normally increase metabolic rate [10]. Consequently, the metabolic rate decreases, eliminating that potential source of heat production.

The hypothalamus also activates sympathetic nerves that supply the sweat glands, creating perspiration on the surface of the skin. Evaporation of sweat reduces skin temperature, thereby cooling the blood that flows through the dilated skin vessels before it returns to the core [7]. As a result of these activities, core and skin

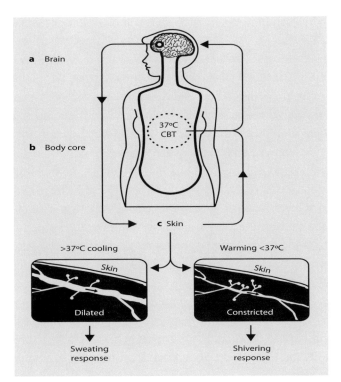

Fig. 2. The temperature circuit with the major control sites that coordinate temperature regulation. **a** Brain includes the hypothalamus. **b** Core body includes the cranial, thoracic and abdominal cavities. **c** Skin, subcutaneous tissue and muscles.

temperature decrease to a specific and well-defined temperature that is commonly termed the body core temperature 'set-point'. In contrast, a decrease in internal body or skin temperature causes responses that decrease heat dissipation [7]. In this case, hypothalamic neurons send signals that result in subcutaneous blood vessel constriction, thereby decreasing blood flow and volume resulting in conserving heat (fig. 2, bottom) from the outer shell. Signals are also sent to the muscles to initiate shivering which is a process that will generate local heat [7]. Consequently, the metabolic rate increases resulting in a source of heat production. As a result of these activities, the internal body cavity and skin temperature increase correcting the initial notification of decreasing core body temperature [7].

Normal functioning of the thermoregulatory circuitry produces a continuous and coordinated response to changes in the internal body temperature [3]. The purpose of these responses is to maintain a constant and consistent internal body cavity temperature that averages 37°C (98.6°F) in a healthy resting adult. This defined core body temperature must be maintained within a narrow range of temperature change in order to maintain optimal function and is commonly referred to as the 'set-point' [11]. A variation in this 'set-point' is influenced by time of day, metabolic rate, physical activity, age and gender. Individual differences considered, the reported overall range of core body temperature taken rectally is 34.4–37.8°C [12]. Nevertheless, regardless of factors that may impact the actual 'set-point' of internal body temperature, the circuitry is responsible for maintaining internal temperature within a narrow 4°C range of temperature fluctuation in order to maintain homeostasis. This temperature range is referred to as the thermal neutral zone and typically maintained with simple and continuous changes in subcutaneous blood flow. Heat-loss or heat-gain mechanisms are only initiated when core body temperature falls outside this zone.

It is thought that VMS results from a malfunction or disruption in the fine balance of the thermoregulatory circuitry resulting in an exaggerated heat-loss response. This exaggerated response initiates an abrupt heat-dissipating mechanism by causing blood vessels to rapidly dilate followed by initiation of the sweating response and decrease in metabolic rate. If these responses result in drastic temperature decreases causing temperatures again to be outside the thermal neutral zone, the heat-gain mechanisms will then be initiated. Blood vessels will rapidly constrict and the shivering response, as in the 'chill' that some patients may feel at the end of a hot flash will be initiated to restore core body temperature with in the 'set-point' range [13]. A true understanding of what causes the thermoregulatory dysfunction that may underlie VMS remains unclear. The next section describes some current hypotheses.

Possible Causes of Temperature Dysfunction

Several hypotheses have suggested that VMS are due to either a malfunction of one or more of the thermoregulatory control mechanisms, a disruption in communication between these mechanisms, or a change in temperature 'set-point' sensitivity. Regardless of which hypothesis is correct, all of them are associated with dysfunction occurring within the three major thermoregulatory sites (brain, internal body core, and skin).

Temperature Dysfunction at the Level of the Brain

As early as the 1960s physicians have been experimenting with brain-active drugs to treat VMS in menopausal women without clearly understanding what controls temperature regulation. It is now known that the hypothalamus is thought to be the primary temperature control center of the brain that is responsible for maintaining temperature regulation. The hypothalamus, along with the limbic region, is responsible for integrating data received from thermal receptors both inside and outside the CNS. This region of the brain functions as the body's 'thermostat'. The hypothalamus is responsible for responding to changes in internal body temperature by initiating and coordinating thermoregulatory mechanisms that will result in either heat generation or dissipation. One way in which this is accomplished is via release of neurotransmitters, which are the chemical messengers of neurotransmission. Two neurotransmitters thought to be involved in communicating and modulating temperature homeostasis in the hypothalamus are serotonin (5-HT), also known as 5-hydroxytryptamine and norepinephrine (NE). It is thought that estrogens can directly and indirectly modulate 5-HT and NE levels in the brain as well as in the hypothalamus [14]. As a result, gonadal hormone changes cause these levels of transmitters to become unstable and inconsistently produced.

In addition, evidence supports the role of gonadal hormones in modulating the function of specific neuroreceptors known to play a role in temperature regulation [15, 16]. Considerable evidence has demonstrated the involvement of the alpha2 [17] and beta [18] adrenergic receptors in temperature regulation. Additionally, both the nicotinic and muscarinic receptors (cholinergic system) have been shown to play a role in modulating the central aspects of temperature [19, 20]. Thus, fluctuations or decline in gonadal hormone levels may affect the physiologically function of these receptors, disrupting the intricate balance necessary to maintain temperature regulation.

Dysfunction in the 'Set-Point' of Core Body Temperature

Another hypothesis focuses on a change in the range (or sensitivity) of the thermal neutral zone. The thermal neutral zone is an established range of temperature that is maintained by simple and continuous changes in subcutaneous blood flow; however, small changes within this zone do not initiate the heat dissipation or generation mechanisms. This suggests that core body temperature is maintained between an upper and lower temperature limit [21, 22]. Heat-dissipation or heat-generation mechanisms require a greater change in internal core body temperature is required. If internal body temperature crosses over the upper temperature threshold, heat-dissipating actions are triggered. Whereas, when core body temperature crosses over the lower temperature threshold, heat-generating mechanisms are triggered [14].

There is some evidence, although limited, that the thermal neutral zone is narrowed during menopause as a result of fluctuating or declining ovarian hormone levels [21, 22]. Under these conditions, even small core body temperature increases will cross the upper or sweating threshold. When this occurs the patient feels an intense flash of heat that triggers the heat-dissipating mechanisms [23, 24]. If there is an exaggerated response that dissipates heat rapidly, over compensation in heat loss occurs and the heat-generation process is then initiated. The final phase in features of severe VMS is that the patient experiences shivering and the sensation of being chilled.

Another potential aspect that may contribute to hormone regulated thermoregulatory dysfunction is changes in the peripheral vasculature and vasculature reactivity [7]. As stated earlier, the skin is an important thermoregulatory control center that is responsible for participating in the mechanisms of heat dissipation and generation. Estrogens act on the vascular system, modulating arteriolar and venous tone to change blood flow patterns that impact blood flow volume [25]. Because estrogens have this peripheral effect, changes in the levels of estrogens can affect vasomotor tone and reaction time and, as a result, may contribute, in part, to the thermoregulatory dysfunction that underlies VMS [3, 25].

Preclinical Animal Models Used to Study Temperature Regulation

The underlying physiology and signaling pathways associated with thermoregulatory dysfunction caused by gonadal hormone changes are currently unknown due to the limited research focus in this therapeutic area. Preclinical rodent models can be utilized to study the impact of ovarian hormones on various systems involved in temperature regulation. These models of thermoregulatory dysfunction are based on measuring changes in tail skin and core body temperature in ovariectomized rats. The models can also be used to evaluate various compounds that target specific systems (i.e. receptors, neurotransmitters, channels and enzymes) and brain regions thought to be involved in temperature regulation. Studying the effects of known pharmacological agents in these models can help to discern the pathways and systems involved, at least in part, in ovarian hormone-dependent temperature regulation. Although these preclinical models lack some degree of validity for menopausal hot flashes, previous studies have demonstrated that they exhibit predictive validity of efficacy in the clinic [26–29]. These models can be used to evaluate the effects of agents on temperature regulation in its entirety and define whether they are impinging specifically on brain function, internal body temperature, or vasculature reactivity.

Treatment of Vasomotor Symptoms

Hormone therapy (HT) has been used effectively to alleviate VMS in postmenopausal women for the past 50 years. Research has focused largely on developing various hormonal combinations and lower dose HT formulations to improve safety and tolerability profiles. In addition to treating VMS associated with menopause, HT also effectively treats symptoms of vaginal atrophy and prevents postmenopausal osteoporosis. Although estrogens and some progestins are able to effectively correct thermoregulatory dysfunction in patients suffering with VMS, the underlying mechanisms by which hormones modulate temperature regulation is not understood.

Various antidepressant, anticonvulsant, sedative and older centrally-acting antihypertensive medications have been investigated for the treatment of VMS in populations for whom HT is contraindicated [3]. These populations include women with a history of breast cancer and men who have undergone androgen ablation therapy for prostate cancer. The most researched agents to date include agents typically used to treat major depressive disorder such as selective serotonin reuptake inhibitors (SSRIs; fluoxetine, citalopram, paroxetine) and dual-acting serotonin norepinephrine reuptake inhibitors (SNRIs; venlafaxine and desvenlafaxine). Because of the proposed role of 5-HT and NE transmitters in thermoregulation, these types of compounds are of particular interest to clinical scientists.

It is clear that the pathophysiology of VMS is not fully understood, and identifying the underlying mechanisms involved in thermoregulation will be important in developing nonhormonal therapies. The relationship between core body temperature and occurrence of hot flashes has been the primary focus of earlier research evaluating the etiology of hot flashes. However, the majority of investigational drugs currently being evaluated for the treatment of VMS are focusing on CNS active agents that modulate neurotransmitters or neuroreceptors rather than modulating changes in the internal core temperature. At this time, there is no evidence to suggest that the mechanisms involved in causing VMS would be different in the various populations (i.e. postmenopausal, non-postmenopausal, cancer survivors, and GnRH-treated patients) experiencing these symptoms.

Conclusion

Although patients have been seeking treatment for VMS for decades, surprisingly little is known about the etiology of this temperature dysfunction. What is known is that hormone-based therapies are effective in alleviating VMS and fluctuating/declining gonadal hormones are thought to be responsible for the onset and persistence of these symptoms. To date in the US, only hormone-based therapies are approved for the treatment of menopause-associated VMS in healthy postmenopausal women. The need to understand the underlying biology and identify the systems that are disrupted due to changes in gonadal hormones are important in order to develop alternative therapies. Additionally, it should be noted that although VMS are thought to be the hallmark of the menopause transition, other symptoms that may be associated with changes in gonadal hormone levels should be assessed. Symptoms such as sleep disturbances, mood disorders, changes in energy level, decreased libido and somatic symptoms should also be evaluated. It is unknown whether these symptoms occur in parallel or as a result of VMS. It is possible that these additional symptoms reported by women during the menopausal transition share a common etiology and shared underlying pathophysiology. Thus, the need to understand the affected biological pathways that are disrupted in patients experiencing VMS during menopause is necessary and may additionally provide understanding of other symptoms reported during this transition period.

References

1 Rodstrom K, Bengtsson C, Lissner L, Milsom I, Sundh V, Bjorkelund C: A longitudinal study of the treatment of hot flushes: the population study of women in Gothenburg during a quarter of a century (comment). Menopause 2002;9:156–161.
2 Feldman BM, Voda A, Gronseth E: The prevalence of hot flash and associated variables among perimenopausal women. Res Nurs Health 1985;8:261–268.
3 Deecher DC: Physiology of thermoregulatory dysfunction and current approaches to the treatment of vasomotor symptoms. Expert Opin Investig Drugs 2005;14:435–448.
4 Land SR, Wickerham DL, Costantino JP, Ritter MW, Vogel VG, Lee M, Pajon ER, Wade JL 3rd, Dakhil S, Lockhart JB Jr, Wolmark N, Ganz PA: Patient-reported symptoms and quality of life during treatment with tamoxifen or raloxifene for breast cancer prevention: the NSABP Study of Tamoxifen and Raloxifene (STAR) P-2 trial. JAMA 2006;295:2742–2751.
5 Mom CH, Buijs C, Willemse PH, Mourits MJ, de Vries EG: Hot flushes in breast cancer patients. Crit Rev Oncol Hematol 2006;57:63–77.
6 Spetz AC, Zetterlund EL, Varenhorst E, Hammar M: Incidence and management of hot flashes in prostate cancer. J Support Oncol 2003;1:263–276.
7 Charkoudian N: Skin blood flow in adult human thermoregulation: how it works, when it does not, and why. Mayo Clin Proc 2003;78:603–612.
8 Boulant JA, Gonzalez RR: The effect of skin temperature on the hypothalamic control of heat loss and heat production. Brain Res 1977;120:367–372.
9 Hensel H: Neural processes in thermoregulation. Physiol Rev 1973;53:948–1017.
10 Huether SE, Leo J: Pain, Temperature Regulation, Sleep, and Sensory Function, ed 4. St. Louis, Mosby, 2002.
11 Guyton AC, Hall JE: Textbook of Medical Physiology, ed 11. Philadelphia, Elsevier Saunders, 2006.
12 Sund-Levander M, Forsberg C, Wahren LK: Normal oral, rectal, tympanic and axillary body temperature in adult men and women: a systematic literature review. Scand J Caring Sci 2002;16:122–128.
13 Kronenberg F: Hot Flashes, ed 2. Philadelphia, Lippincott Williams & Wilkins, 1999.
14 Deecher DC, Dorries K: Understanding the pathophysiology of vasomotor symptoms (hot flushes and night sweats) that occur in perimenopause, menopause, and postmenopause life stages. Arch Womens Ment Health 2007;10:247–257.
15 Klangkalya B, Chan A: The effects of ovarian hormones on beta-adrenergic and muscarinic receptors in rat heart. Life Sci 1988;42:2307–2314.
16 Smith YR, Minoshima S, Kuhl DE, Zubieta JK: Effects of long-term hormone therapy on cholinergic synaptic concentrations in healthy postmenopausal women. J Clin Endocrinol Metab 2001;86:679–684.
17 Katovich MJ, Simpkins JW, Barney CC: Alpha-adrenergic mediation of the tail skin temperature response to naloxone in morphine-dependent rats. Brain Res 1987;426:55–61.
18 Mogilnicka E, Klimek V, Nowak G, Czyrak A: Clonidine and a beta-agonists induce hyperthermia in rats at high ambient temperature. J Neural Transm Gen Sect 1985;63:223–235.
19 Lin MT, Chen FF, Chern YF, Fung TC: The role of the cholinergic system in the central control of thermoregulation in rats. Can J Physiol Pharmacol 1979;57:1205–1212.
20 Saxena AK, Tangri KK, Mishra N, Vrat S, Bhargava KP: Presence of cholinoceptors in mesencephalic raphe nuclei concerned in thermoregulation in rabbits. Clin Exp Pharmacol Physiol 1984;11:105–110.
21 Freedman RR, Krell W: Reduced thermoregulatory null zone in postmenopausal women with hot flashes. Am J Obstet Gynecol 1999;181:66–70.
22 Freedman RR: Hot flashes: behavioral treatments, mechanisms, and relation to sleep. Am J Med 2005;118:124–130.
23 Shanafelt TD, Barton DL, Adjei AA, Loprinzi CL: Pathophysiology and treatment of hot flashes. Mayo Clinic Proc 2002;77:1207–1218.
24 Freedman RR: Pathophysiology and treatment of menopausal hot flashes. Semin Reprod Med 2005;23:117–125.

25 Kronenberg F: Hot flashes: epidemiology and physiology. Ann NY Acad Sci 1990;592:52–86; discussion 123–133.

26 Simpkins JW, Katovich MJ, Song IC: Similarities between morphine withdrawal in the rat and the menopausal hot flush. Life Sci 1983;32:1957–1966.

27 Berendsen HHG, Weekers AHJ, Kloosterboer HJ: Effect of tibolone and raloxifene on the tail temperature of oestrogen-deficient rats. Eur J Pharmacol 2001;419:47–54.

28 Sipe K, Leventhal L, Burroughs K, Cosmi S, Johnston GH, Deecher DC: Serotonin 2A receptors modulate tail-skin temperature in two rodent models of estrogen deficiency-related thermoregulatory dysfunction. Brain Res 2004;1028:191–202.

29 Deecher DC, Alfinito PD, Leventhal L, Cosmi S, Johnston GH, Merchenthaler I, Winneker R: Alleviation of thermoregulatory dysfunction with the new serotonin and norepinephrine reuptake inhibitor desvenlafaxine succinate in ovariectomized rodent models. Endocrinology 2007;148:1376–1383.

Darlene C. Deecher, PhD
Women's Health, Wyeth Research
500 Arcola Road RN3164
Collegeville, PA 19426 (USA)
Tel. +1 215 529 7935, E-Mail ddeecher@comcast.net

Soares CN, Warren M (eds): The Menopausal Transition. Interface between Gynecology and Psychiatry.
Key Issues in Mental Health. Basel, Karger, 2009, vol 175, pp 88–101

Hormone Dynamics and Menopausal Symptoms: The Clinical Role of Vasomotor Symptoms and Sleep Disturbances

Robert R. Freedman

Departments of Psychiatry and Obstetrics and Gynecology, Detroit, Mich., USA

Abstract

Hot flashes are the most common symptom associated with menopause, although prevalence estimates are lower in some rural and non-Western areas. The symptoms are characteristic of a heat-dissipation response and consist of sweating on the face, neck, and chest, as well as peripheral vasodilation. Although hot flashes clearly accompany the estrogen withdrawal at menopause, estrogen alone is not responsible, because levels do not differ between symptomatic and asymptomatic women. Until recently, it was thought that hot flashes were triggered by a sudden, downward resetting of the hypothalamic set point, because there was no evidence of increased core body temperature. However, we recently obtained such evidence, using a rapidly responding ingested telemetry pill. We then found that the thermoneutral zone, within which sweating, peripheral vasodilation, and shivering do not occur, is virtually nonexistent in symptomatic women, but normal (about 0.4°C) in asymptomatic women. Thus, we believe that small temperature elevations preceding hot flashes acting within a reduced thermoneutral zone constitute the triggering mechanism. We also demonstrate that central sympathetic activation is elevated in symptomatic women, which, in animal studies, reduces the thermoneutral zone. Clonidine reduces central sympathetic activation, widens the thermoneutral zone, and ameliorates hot flashes. Estrogen virtually eliminates hot flashes and widens the thermoneutral zone, but the pathway through which this occurs is not known. Behavioral relaxation procedures reduce hot flash frequency to the same extent as clonidine (about 50%), but their mechanism of action is also not understood.

Hot flashes are the most common symptom of the climacteric and occur in most post-menopausal and many perimenopausal women [1]. Hot flash prevalence among naturally menopausal women has been reported to be 68–82% in the United States [2], 60% in Sweden [3], and 62% in Australia [4]. The median age of onset is about 51 years [5]. Among ovariectomized women, the prevalence of hot flashes is approximately 90% [2]. Feldman et al. [2] found that 64% of women reported hot flashes for 1–5 years and Kronenberg [5] found the median length of the symptomatic period to be 4 years.

Research conducted by the author supported by NIH Merit Award, R37-AG05233 and by NIH MH-68683.

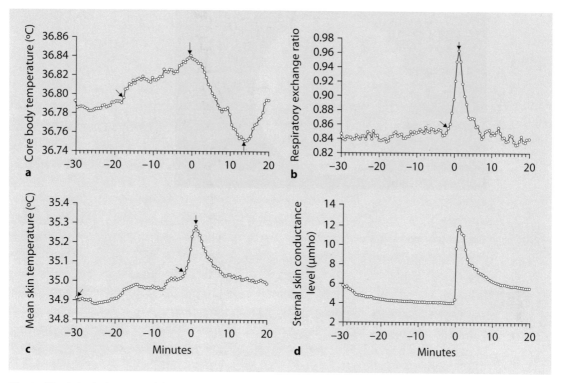

Fig. 1. Physiological events of the hot flash. **a** Core body temperature (means) during menopausal hot flashes. **b** Respiratory exchange ratio (means) during hot flashes. **c** Mean skin temperature (means) during hot flashes. **d** Sternal skin conductance (means) during hot flashes. Time 0 is the beginning of the sternal skin conductance response. Intervals between arrows are significantly different from each other at $p < 0.05$, Duncan's test.

Hot Flash Physiology

Hot flashes are generally described as internal sensations of intense heat, accompanied by sweating, chills, and clamminess. They usually last from about 1 to 5 min, but occasionally much longer. Sweating usually occurs superior to the sternum, but rarely in the lower body.

A hot flash is an exaggerated heat dissipation response. Therefore, peripheral vasodilation, evidenced by increased skin temperature and blood flow, occurs in all areas that have been measured, including the digits, hand, cheek, forehead, arm, leg, and abdomen [6–10].

Sweating and its electrical analog, skin conductance, increase during hot flashes. We simultaneously recorded these measures during 29 hot flashes in 14 women [6]. There was a close temporal correspondence between both measures and both increased significantly. Measurable sweating occurred in 90% of the flashes (fig. 1).

Increased sternal skin conductance has proved to be the best objective marker of hot flashes. An increase in this measure ≥2 μmho/30 s corresponded with 95 [11], 90

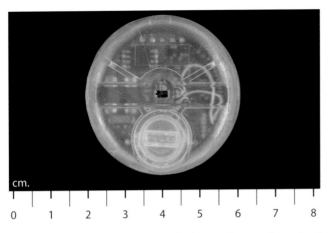

Fig. 2. Miniature, hygrometric hot flash recorder. Weight = 14 g. Scale in cm.

[12], and 80% [13] of self-reported hot flashes. No such responses were recorded in premenopausal or asymptomatic postmenopausal women [11, 12].

The skin conductance measurement is particularly useful for treatment studies, because it can be recorded outside the laboratory over long periods of time and does not require the patient's intervention. Using the same recording methods with ambulatory monitors, we found an 86% coincidence between the skin conductance criterion (2 µmho/30 s) and patient event marks [11]. A second study found an agreement rate of 77% [12].

More recently, a miniature hot flash recorder using neither electrodes nor gel, which must be changed daily, was invented by the author (fig. 2) [14]. The device uses a relative humidity (RH) sensor and attaches over the sternum with double-sided adhesive collars. It weighs 14 g and records for 1 month on a single hearing aid battery [7]. In 10 symptomatic women recorded in the laboratory, the agreement among an RH increase ≥3%/min, a skin conductance increase ≥2 µmho/30 s, and a patient-activated event marker were 100%. In the field, using skin conductance as the gold standard, the sensitivity was 90.9%, the specificity was 95.2%, and the positive predictive value (PPV) was 95.6%. Using the event marks as the gold standard, the PPV for RH was 59.7%. Thus, hot flashes are vastly underreported compared to objective, physiological methods.

Endocrinology of Hot Flashes

Since hot flashes accompany the estrogen withdrawal at menopause, there is little doubt that estrogens play a role in their initiation. This is supported by the fact that estrogen administration virtually eliminates hot flashes [15]. However, estrogen reduction alone does not explain their etiology, because there are no correlations between hot flash occurrence and plasma [16], urinary [17], or vaginal [18] levels of estrogens, nor are there differences in plasma levels in women with and without hot flashes [19, 20]. Additionally, clonidine reduces hot flash frequency without changing circulating estrogen levels [21] and prepubertal girls have low estrogen levels, but no hot flashes. Thus, estrogen withdrawal is necessary but not sufficient to explain the occurrence of hot flashes.

Because gonadotropins become elevated at menopause, their role in the etiology of hot flashes was investigated. First, a temporal correspondence between LH (lutenizing hormone) pulses and hot flashes was reported [22, 23]. However, it was subsequently found that women with isolated gonadotropin deficiency had hot flashes but no LH pulses, and women with hypothalamic amenorrhea had LH pulses but no hot flashes [24]. Furthermore, hot flashes occur in hypophysectomized women who have no LH pulses [25], in women with pituitary insufficiency and hypoestrogenism [26], and in women with LH release suppressed by gonadotropin-release hormone administration [27, 28]. Thus, LH pulses are not the basis for hot flashes.

Next, an opioidergic system was considered in the etiology of hot flashes. Lightman et al. [29] found that naloxone infusion reduced hot flashes and LH pulses in 6 symptomatic women, but subsequent attempts to replicate this failed [30]. Tepper et al. [31] found that plasma β-endorphin concentrations decreased significantly before hot flashes, whereas, Genazzani et al. [32] found the opposite effect. Thus, there is no consistent evidence of the involvement of an opiodergic system in hot flashes.

There is considerable evidence from animal studies that norepinephrine plays an important role in thermoregulation, mediated, in part, by α_2-adrenergic receptors [33]. Injection of norepinephrine into the preoptic hypothalamus of rabbits causes peripheral vasodilation and heat loss, followed by a decline in core body temperature (T_c) [33]. Also, there is evidence that gonadal steroids modulate α_2-adrenergic receptors [34]. Although plasma norepinephrine levels do not increase before or during hot flashes [5], these do not reflect levels in the brain [35]. We therefore studied plasma MHPG (3-methoxy-4-hydroxyphenylglycol), which was initially thought to be representative of brain levels. We found that basal levels of this compound were significantly higher in symptomatic versus asymptomatic women, and increased significantly further during hot flashes [36].

However, approximately 50% of free MHPG that enters the blood is metabolized peripherally to VMA (varillylmandelic acid), which competes with MHPG production [35]. We therefore measured MHPG and VMA before and during hot flashes in 14 symptomatic women [6]. We replicated our previous finding that MHPG increases during hot flashes and also found that VMA did not change, consistent with a central origin for MHPG. However, more recent work [37] showed that only a minority of plasma MHPG is derived from the brain, with the majority coming from skeletal muscle. Therefore, MHPG can only be used to reflect whole-body sympathetic activation.

The most convincing evidence that central noradrenergic activation is involved in the etiology of hot flashes comes from clinical studies. It had already been shown that clonidine, an α_2-adrenergic agonist that reduces brain norepinephrine, significantly reduces hot flash frequency [21]. In a controlled laboratory investigation, we then showed that yohimbine, an α_2-adrenergic antagonist that elevates brain NE [37], provoked hot flashes in symptomatic women, whereas clonidine ameliorated them [38]. These data support the theory that elevated brain NE acting at central α_2-adrenoceptors is involved in the initiation of hot flashes. Postmortem studies have shown that most α_2-receptors in the human brain are inhibitory, presynaptic receptors [39]. Blockade of these receptors with yohimbine would increase NE release, whereas clonidine would have the opposite effect [40, 41]. Thus, the yohimbine provocation and clonidine inhibition of hot flashes may reflect a deficit in inhibitory α_2-receptor function in symptomatic women. Given that estrogens modulate brain adrenergic receptors [42, 43], it is possible that the estrogen withdrawal at menopause is associated with this deficit.

Thermoregulation and Hot Flashes

Normal thermoregulation occurs between upper thresholds for sweating and peripheral vasodilation and lower thresholds for peripheral vasoconstriction and shivering. If T_c were elevated in women with hot flashes, their symptoms of sweating and peripheral vasodilation could be explained. Early studies used measurements of rectal and esophageal temperature [44] and did not find this effect. However, these methods have long thermal lag times and may have been too slow to capture the T_c elevations.

We therefore measured T_c using an ingested radiotelemetry pill, which responds more rapidly than the esophageal and rectal methods. Defining hot flashes using the sternal skin conductance response, we found small but statistically significant T_c elevations preceding the majority of flashes [19]. We replicated these findings in two subsequent studies, in which we found that significant T_c elevations preceded 76% (fig. 1) [6] and 65% [45] of the flashes, respectively. Rectal temperature did not significantly change [45].

The T_c elevations could be caused by increased metabolic rate (heat production) and/or peripheral vasoconstriction (decreased heat loss). We indeed found significant increases in metabolic rate, but they were simultaneous with peripheral vasodilation and sweating; peripheral vasoconstriction did not occur (fig. 1) [6]. Therefore, the T_c elevations are not driven by metabolic rate. Modest increases in heart rate, approximately 7–15 beats/min, do not coincide with the increases in metabolic rate [7, 8].

As stated above, T_c in homeotherms is regulated between upper thresholds for sweating and peripheral vasodilation and lower thresholds for peripheral vasoconstriction and shivering. Between these thresholds is a neutral zone within which major thermoregulatory adjustments (sweating and shivering) [46] do not occur. Fine thermoregulatory adjustments within this zone are made by variations in peripheral

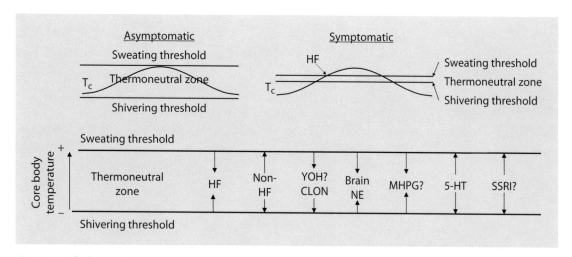

Fig. 3. Hot flash model. Small core body temperature (Tc) elevations acting within a reduced thermoneutral zone trigger HFs in symptomatic postmenopausal women. We have shown that the thermoneutral zone is narrowed in symptomatic women. Elevated brain norepinephrine (NE) in animals reduces this zone. Yohimbine (YOH) elevates brain norepinephrine and should reduce this zone. Conversely, clonidine (CLON) should widen it. HF = Symptomatic women; non-HF = asymptomatic women; MHPG = 3-methoxy-4-hydroxyphenylglycol (the primary NE metabolite); 5-HT = serotonin; SSRI = selective serotonin reuptake inhibitor.

blood flow. Having found T_c elevations preceding hot flashes, we reasoned that the width of the thermoneutral zone in women with hot flashes might be narrowed.

We then performed a study in which we measured the thermoneutral zone in symptomatic and asymptomatic postmenopausal women using ambient heating and cooling. We measured T_c using a rectal probe and the ingested radiotelemetry pill and determined the sweating and shivering thresholds for each [20]. In a subsequent session, we increased T_c to the sweating threshold using exercise. We measured the thermoneutral zone (by both methods) to be 0.0°C in the asymptomatic women. The T_c sweating thresholds were the same for heating and exercise and were accompanied by objective and subjective hot flashes in every case. Sweat rates in the symptomatic women were twice those of the asymptomatic women (p < 0.05). No hot flashes occurred in the asymptomatic women.

Thus, we believe that hot flashes are triggered by T_c elevations acting within a greatly reduced thermoneutral zone in symptomatic postmenopausal women (fig. 3). A hot flash, consisting of sweating and peripheral vasodilation, is triggered when T_c reaches the upper threshold. T_c then declines, and when the lower threshold is crossed, shivering occurs. In a subsequent study, we found that the T_c elevations also occur in asymptomatic women [47]. Therefore, the critical factor in the etiology of hot flashes is the narrowing of the thermoneutral zone. What accounts for this?

Animal studies have shown that increased brain NE narrows the width of the thermoneutral zone [33]. Conversely, clonidine reduces NE release, increases the sweating

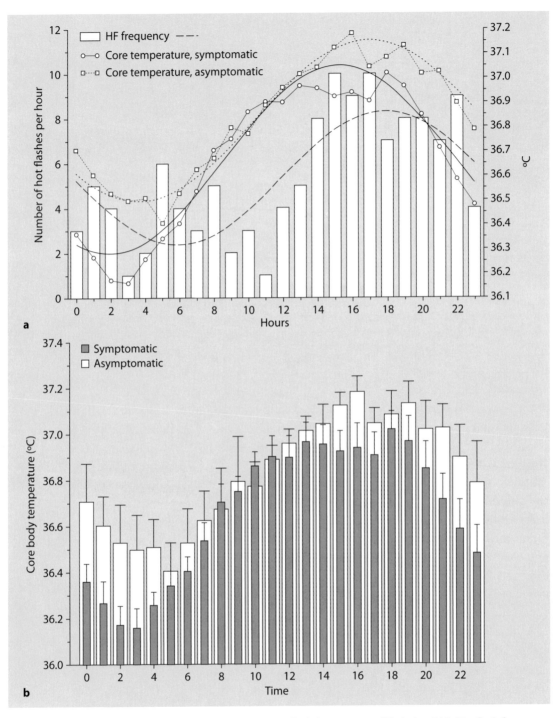

Fig. 4. Circadian rhythm of hot flashes. **a** Hot-flash frequency and T_c during 24 h. Hot flash frequency in 10 symptomatic women (bars); best-fit cosine curve for hot flash frequency (dashed line); 24-hour T_c data for 10 symptomatic women (■) with best-fit cosine (solid line); 24-hour T_c data in 6 asymptomatic women (□) with best-fit cosine curve (dotted line). **b** 24-hour T_c (mean ± SE) in symptomatic and asymptomatic women.

threshold, and lowers the shivering threshold. Thus, we suggest that elevated brain NE narrows the thermoregulatory interthreshold zone in symptomatic postmenopausal women (fig. 4).

Since clonidine has been shown to ameliorate hot flashes [21], we decided to study its effects on the thermoneutral zone. Since most of the narrowing found in our previous study was due to depression of the sweating threshold, we did not measure the shivering threshold in this study. We found that clonidine significantly raised the sweating threshold in women with hot flashes, whereas, the opposite effect was obtained in asymptomatic women. Thus, we believe that clonidine ameliorates hot flashes by elevation of the T_c sweating threshold.

Since estrogen is the most effective treatment for hot flashes, we decided to study its effects upon the sweating threshold. Women reporting at least 6 hot flashes/day were randomly assigned to receive 1 mg/day p.o., 17β-estradiol (n = 12) or placebo (n = 12) for 90 days. Hot flashes were objectively measured in the laboratory before and after treatment along with T_c elevations, plasma MHPG, and the T_c sweating threshold. In the treated group, hot flash frequency was significantly reduced by ~65% and the T_c sweating threshold significantly elevated. These effects did not occur in the placebo group. MHPG did not significantly change in either group. Thus, we believe that estrogen ameliorates hot flashes by raising the T_c sweating threshold although the details of this mechanism are not yet known.

Circadian Rhythms

The circadian rhythm of T_c is well known, and similar variations in other thermoregulatory parameters, such as heat conductance and sweating, have also been shown. These patterns suggest that the thermoregulatory effector responses of hot flashes might also demonstrate temporal variations. A previous study showed circadian rhythmicity of self-reported hot flashes in some menopausal women, but no physiologic data were collected [48]. We recruited and screened 10 symptomatic and 6 asymptomatic postmenopausal women [19]. Each received 24-hour ambulatory monitoring of sternal skin conductance level to detect hot flashes as well as ambient temperature, skin temperature and T_c. The last measure was recorded using the ingested radiotelemetry pill. Cosinor analysis demonstrated a circadian rhythm (p < 0.02) of hot flashes with a peak around 1,825 h (fig. 4). This rhythm lagged the circadian rhythm of T_c in symptomatic women by about 3 h. T_c values of the symptomatic women were lower than those of the asymptomatic women (p < 0.05) from 00.00 to 04.00 and at 15.00 and 22.00 h. The majority of hot flashes were preceded by elevations in T_c, a statistically significant effect (p < 0.05). Hot flashes began at significantly (p < 0.02) higher levels of T_c (36.82 ± 0.04°C) compared with all non-flash periods (36.70 ± 0.005°C). These data are consistent with the hypothesis that elevated T_c serves as part of the hot flash triggering mechanism.

Table 1. Do hot flashes and sleep disturbance occur with menopause?

Study	Type	Self-reported HFs	Sleep disturbance
McKinlay [49]	cross-sectional	+	+
Bungay et al. [50]	cross-sectional	+	+
Hunter [51]	cross-sectional	+	+
Matthews [52]	longitudinal	+	–
Hunter [53]	cross-sectional	+	+
Holte [54]	longitudinal	+	–
Shaver [55]	cross-sectional	+	–
McKinlay [56]	longitudinal	+	+
Kuh et al. [57]	longitudinal	+	+
Kravitz [58]	longitudinal	+	+

Sleep Disturbance and Menopause

Disturbed sleep has been reported in the majority of descriptive studies of menopause (table 1), and it is generally assumed that this is due to hot flashes (HFs). However, recent studies conducted in our laboratory and others have called this relationship into question. It is the purpose of this section to briefly review the occurrence of sleep disturbance in menopause, the role of HFs in this disturbance, and the effects of estrogen upon it.

In our first investigation [59], we found no significant differences among age-matched cycling women, asymptomatic postmenopausal women, and symptomatic postmenopausal women on any physiological or self-reported sleep measure, on the Multiple Sleep Latency Test (MSLT), or on any performance or psychological test. Moreover, physiological HF recordings showed that these tended to occur after rather than before arousals and awakenings. If HFs were producing the arousals and awakenings, one would have expected the HFs to occur first.

This relationship was further elucidated in our second investigation [60]. Because REM sleep suppresses thermoregulatory effector responses (such as HFs) [61] and is more frequent in the second half of the night, we analyzed the data by halves of the night. Here, we found that in the first half of the night, the HFs did precede the arousals and awakenings, whereas in the second half of the night this order was reversed. Thus, it is possible that in the first half of the night, HFs are producing objective sleep disturbance, the first such evidence reported.

The findings of our first study are supported by those of the Wisconsin Sleep Cohort Study [62] which measured sleep quality by complete laboratory polysomnography

(PSG) and by self-reports in a probability sample of 589 pre-, peri-, and postmeno-pausal women. Sleep quality was not worse in peri- or postmenopausal women nor in symptomatic versus asymptomatic women on any physiological measure. This study did find significant elevations in reported sleep dissatisfaction in post- versus pre-menopausal, and peri- versus premenopausal women.

More recently, we completed a study in which 102 women, ages 44–56 years, com-plaining of poor sleep were recorded in the laboratory [63]. They were also assessed with the Pittsburgh Sleep Quality Index (PSQI) [64] and with the Hamilton Depression and Anxiety scales. We found that 53% of the women had apnea, restless legs, or both. The best predictors of objective sleep quality (laboratory sleep efficiency) were apneas, periodic limb movements, and arousals. The best predictors of subjective sleep qual-ity (PSQI total score) were the Hamilton anxiety score and the number of hot flashes in the first half of the night. Thus, primary sleep disorders (apnea and restless legs syndrome) are common in midlife women. Amelioration of hot flashes may reduce some complaints of poor sleep, but will not necessarily alleviate underlying primary sleep disorders. Because these can result in significant morbidity and mortality, they require careful attention in peri- and postmenopausal women.

Estrogen and Sleep

There are seven published studies of the effects of estrogen on laboratory-recorded sleep, although different studies reported different measures. Table 2 shows that some studies reported decreased wake time and arousals, whereas one found decreased sleep latency. Three studies found increased REM sleep. Interestingly, the single study reporting no objective sleep improvement recorded subjects at an ambient tempera-ture of 16°C [65]. Previous research showed that hot flashes are suppressed at ambi-ent temperatures <19°C [60, 63]. Half of the studies in table 2 found that estrogen improved subjective sleep quality, whereas half did not. No study used an objective assessment of sleepiness, such as the Multiple Sleep Latency Test (MSLT).

Sleep disorders are relatively common in peri- and postmenopausal women. Although complaints of poor sleep in this population are often attributed to the effects of hot flashes, this is often not the case. We, and others, have shown that apnea and restless legs syndrome are common in these women. Women suspected of having sleep apnea, i.e. obese women who snore and have a large neck circumference, should be referred to a sleep disorders center accredited by the American Sleep Disorders Association (ASDA) for evaluation and treatment. Women complaining of periodic limb movements should be referred in the same manner.

As shown earlier, the effects of estrogens on sleep are equivocal. Women com-plaining of hot flash-induced sleep disturbance should first be instructed to reduce the ambient temperature to 64°F for the first 4 h of sleep, since this will suppress hot flashes. If this is not effective, pharmacologic treatments should be considered.

Table 2. Effects of estrogen on hot flashes and sleep

Study	HFs	Objective sleep	Subjective sleep
Thomson [65]	no difference	↓ wake time, ↓ arousals ↑ REM	no difference
Schiff [66]	↓	↓ sleep latency, ↑ REM	no difference
Erlik [67]	↓	↓ awakenings	not done
Purdie [68]	↓	no difference (room at 16°C)	no difference
Scharf [69]	↓	↓ awakenings and stage changes ↑ sleep efficiency (no control group)	↑ sleep quality
Polo Kantola [70, 71]	↓	↓ movement arousals ↑ alpha arousals	↑ sleep quality
Antonijevic [72]	not done	↓ wake time, ↑ REM	↑ sleep quality

Our most recent sleep study [63] raised the question of the possible relationships between emotions and sleep in midlife women. A large population-based study by Freeman et al. [73] found a strong association between anxiety and hot flashes. Two subsequent studies [74, 75] by the same group found substantial associations between menopausal status and new [74] and existing [75] depression. Further research on this topic would be of great interest.

References

1 Neugarten BL, Kraines RJ: 'Menopausal symptoms' in women of various ages. Psychosom Med 1965; 27:266–273.
2 Feldman BM, Voda A, Gronseth E: The prevalence of hot flash and associated variables among perimenopausal women. Res Nurs Hlth 1985;8:261–268.
3 Hagstad A, Janson PO: The epidemiology of climacteric symptoms. Acta Obstet Gynecol Scand Suppl 1986;134:59–65.
4 Guthrie JR, Dennerstein L, Hopper JL, Burger HG: Hot flushes, menstrual status, and hormone levels in a population-based sample of midlife women. Obstet Gynecol 1996;88:437–442.
5 Kronenberg F: Hot flashes: epidemiology and physiology. Ann NY Acad Sci 1990;592:52–86.
6 Freedman RR: Biochemical, metabolic, and vascular mechanism in menopausal hot flushes. Fertil Steril 1998;70:1–6.
7 Molnar GW: Body temperature during menopausal hot flashes. J Appl Physiol: Respir Environ Exercise Physiol 1975;38:499–503.
8 Kronenberg F, Cote LJ, Linkie DM, Dyrenfurth I, Downey JA: Menopausal hot flashes: thermoregulatory, cardiovascular, and circulating catecholamine and LH changes. Maturitas 1984;6:31–43.
9 Tataryn IV, Lomax P, Bajorek JG, Chesarek W, Meldrum DR, Judd HL: Postmenopausal hot flushes: a disorder of thermoregulation. Maturitas 1980;2:101–107.
10 Ginsburg J, Swinhoe J, O'Reilly B: Cardiovascular responses during the menopausal hot flush. Br J Obstet Gynaecol 1981;88:925–930.
11 Freedman RR: Laboratory and ambulatory monitoring of menopausal hot flashes. Psychophysiology 1989;26:573–579.

12 Freedman RR, Woodward S, Norton D: Laboratory and ambulatory monitoring of menopausal hot flushes: comparison of symptomatic and asymptomatic women. J Psychophysiol 1992;6:162–166.

13 de Bakker IPM, Everaerd W: Measurement of menopausal hot flushes: validation and cross-validation. Maturitas 25:87–98.

14 Freedman RR, Wasson S: Miniature hygrometric hot flash recorder. Fertil Steril 2007;88:494–496.

15 Kenenmans P, Barentsen R, Van de Weijer P: Practical HRT. Medical Forum International, ed 2, 1996, pp 11–18.

16 Askel S, Schomberg DW, Tyrey L, Hammond CB: Vasomotor symptoms, serum estrogens, gonadotropin levels in surgical menopause. Am J Obstet Gynecol 1976;126:165–169.

17 Stone SC, Mickal A, Rye F, Rye PH: Postmenopausal symptomatology, maturation index, and plasma estrogen levels. Obstet Gynecol 1975;45:625–627.

18 Hutton JD, Jacobs HS, Murray MAF, James VHT: Relation between plasma esterone and estradiol and climacteric symptoms. Lancet 1978;i:678–681.

19 Freedman RR, Norton D, Woodward S, Cornelissen G: Core body temperature and circadian rhythm of hot flashes in menopausal women. J Clin Endocrinol Metab 1995;80:2354–2358.

20 Freedman RR, Krell W: Reduced thermoregulatory null zone in postmenopausal women with hot flashes. Am J Obstet Gynecol 1999;181:66–70.

21 Schindler AE, Muller D, Keller F, Goser R, Runkel F: Studies with clonidine (Dixarit) in menopausal women. Arch Gynecol 1979;227:341–347.

22 Casper RF, Yen SSC, Wilkes MM: Menopausal flushes: a neuroendocrine link with pulsatile luteinzing hormone secretion. Science 1979;205:823–825.

23 Tataryn IV, Meldrum DR, Lu KH, Frumar AM, Judd HL: LH, FSH, and skin temperature during menopausal hot flush. J Clin Endocrinol Metab 1979;49:152–154.

24 Gambone J, Meldrum DR, Laufer L, et al: Further delineation of nypothalamic dysfunction responsible for menopausal hot flashes. J Clin Endocrinol Metab 1984;59:1092–1102.

25 Mulley G, Mitchell RA, Tattersall RB: Hot flushes after hypophysectomy. Br Med J 1977;2:1062.

26 Meldrum DR, Erlik Y, Lu JKH, Judd HL: Objectively recorded hot flushes in patients with pituitary insufficiency. J Clin Endocrinol Metab 1981;52:684–687.

27 Casper RF, Yen SSC: Menopausal flushes: effect of pituitary gonadotropin desensitization by a potent luteinizing hormone releasing factor agonist. J Clin Endocrinol Metab1981;53:1056–1058.

28 DeFazio J, Meldrum DR, Laufer L, et al: Induction of hot flashes in premenopausal women treated with a long-acting GnRH agonist. J Clin Endocrinol Metab 1983;56:445–448.

29 Lightman SL, Jacobs HS, Maguire AK, McGarrick G, Jeffcoate SL: Climacteric flushing: clinical and endocrine response to infusion of naloxone. Br J Obstet Gynaecol 1981;88:919–924.

30 DeFazio J, Verheugen C, Chetkowski R, et al: The effects of naloxone on hot flashes and gonadotropin secretion in postmenopausal women. J Clin Endocrinol Metab 1984;58:578–581.

31 Tepper R, Neri A, Kaufman H, Schoenfield A, Ovadia J: Menopausal hot flushes and plasma β-endorphins. Obstet Gynecol 1987;70:150–152.

32 Genazzani AR, Petraglia F, Facchinetti F, et al: Increase of proopiomelanocortin-related peptides during subjective menopausal flushes. Am J Obstet Gynecol 1984;149:775–779.

33 Bruck K, Zeisberger E: Adaptive changes in thermoregulation and their neuropharmacological basis; in Schonbaum E, Lomax P (eds): Thermoregulation: Physiology and Biochemistry. New York, Pergamon Press, 1990, pp 255–307.

34 Insel PA, Motulskey HJ: Physiologic and pharmacologic regulation of adrenergic receptors; in Insel PA (ed): Adrenergic Receptors in Man. New York, Marcel Dekker, 1987, pp 201–236.

35 Kopin IJ, Blombery P, Ebert MH, et al: Disposition and metabolism ofMHPG-CD$_3$ in humans: plasma MHPG as the principal pathway of norepinephrine metabolism and as an important determinant of CSF levels of MHPG; in Usdin E (ed): Frontiers in Biochemical and Pharmacological Research in Depression. New York, Raven Press, 1984, pp 57–68.

36 Freedman RR, Woodward S: Elevated α$_2$-adrenergic responsiveness in menopausal hot flushes: pharmacologic and biochemical studies; in Lomax P, Schonbaum E (eds): Thermoregulation: The Pathophysiological Basis of Clinical Disorders. Basel, Karger, 1992, pp 6–9.

37 Lambert GW, Kaye DM, Vaz M, et al: Regional origins of 3-methoxy-r-hydroxy-phenylglycol in plasma: effects of chronic sympathetic nervous activation and devervation, and acute reflex sympathetic stimulation. J Auto Nerv Sys 1995;55:169–178.

38 Freedman RR, Woodward S, Sabharwal SC: Adrenergic mechanism in menopausal hot flushes. Obstet Gynecol 1990;76:573–578.

39 Sastre M, Garcia-Sevilla JA: Density of alpha-2A adrenoceptors and Gi proteins in the human brain: ratio of high-affinity agonist to antagonist sites and effect of age. J Pharmacol Exp Ther 1994;269:1062–1072.

40 Starke K, Gothert M, Kilbringer H: Modulation of neurotransmitter release of presynaptic autoreceptors. Physiol Rev 1989;69:864–989.

41 Charney DS, Heninger GR, Sternberg DE: Assessment of α_2-adrenergic autoreceptor function in humans: effects of oral yohimbine. Life Sci 1982;30:2033–2041.

42 Etgen AM, Ansonoff MA, Quesada A: Mechanisms of ovarian steroid regulation of norepinephrine receptor-mediated signal transduction in the hypothalamus: implications for female reproductive physiology. Horm Behav 2001;40:169–177.

43 Ansonoff MA, Etgen AM: Receptor phosphoylation mediates estradiol reduction of alpha 2-adrenoceptor coupling to G protein in the hypothalamus of female rats. Endocrine 2001;14:165–174.

44 Freedman RR, Woodward S: Core body temperature during menopausal hot flashes. Fertil Steril 1996;65:1141–1149.

45 Freedman RR, Norton D, Woodward S, Cornelissen G: Core body temperature and circadian rhythm of hot flashes in menopausal women. J Clin Endocrinol Metab 1995;80:2354–2358.

46 Savage MV, Brengelmann GL: Control of skin blood flow in the neutral zone of human temperature regulation. J Appl Physiol 1996;80:1249–1257.

47 Freedman RR: Core body temperature variation in symptomatic and asymptomatic postmenopausal women: brief report. Menopause 2002;9:399–401.

48 Albright DL, Voda AM, Smolensky MH, Hsi B, Decker M: Circadian rhythms in hot flashes in natural and surgically induced menopause. Chronobiol Internat 1989;6:279–284.

49 McKinlay SM, Jefferys M: The menopause syndrome. Br J Prev Soc Med 1974;28:108–115.

50 Bungay GT, Vessey MP, McPherson CK: Study of symptoms in middle life with special reference to the menopause. BMJ 1980;19:181–183.

51 Hunter M, Battersby R, Whitehead M: Relationships between psychological symptoms, somatic complaints and menopausal status. Maturitas 1986;8:217–228.

52 Matthews KA, Wing RR, Kuller LH, Meilahn EN, Kelsey SF: Influences of natural menopause on psychological characteristics and symptoms of middle-aged healthy women. J Consult Clin Psychol 1990;38:345–351.

53 Hunter M: The south-east England longitudinal study of the climacteric and postmenopause. Maturitas 1992;14:117–126.

54 Holte A: Influences of natural menopause on health complaints: a prospective study of healthy Norwegian women. Maturitas 1992;127–141.

55 Shaver JLF, Paulsen VM: Sleep, psychological distress, and somatic symptoms in perimenopausal women. Farm Pract Res J 1993;13:373–384.

56 Avis NE, Brambilla D, McKinlay SM, Vass K: A longitudinal analysis of the association between menopause and depression. Ann Epidemiol 1994;4:214–220.

57 Kuh DL, Wadsworth M, Hardy R: Women's health in midlife: the influence of the menopause, social factors and health in earlier life. Br J Obstet Gynaecol 1997;104:923–933.

58 Kravitz HM, Ganz PA, Bromberger J, Powell LH, Sutton-Tyrrell K, Meyer PM: Sleep difficulty in women at midlife: a community survey of sleep and the menopausal transition. Menopause 2003;10:19–28.

59 Freedman RR, Roehrs TA: Lack of sleep disturbance from menopausal hot flashes. Fertil Steril 2004;82:138–144.

60 Freedman RR, Roehers TA: Effects of REM sleep and ambient temperature on hot flash-induced sleep disturbance. Menopause 2006;13:576–583.

61 Parmeggiani PL, Zamboni G, Cianci T, Calasso M: Absence of thermoregulatory vasomotor responses during fast wave sleep in cats. Electroencephalogr Clin Neurophysiol 1977;42:372–380.

62 Young T, Rabago D, Zgierska A, Austin D, Finn L: Objective and subjective sleep quality in premenopausal, perimenopausal, and postmenopausal women in the Wisconsin cohort study. Sleep 2003;26:677–672.

63 Freedman RR, Roehrs TA: Sleep disturbance in menopause. Menopause 2007;14:826–829.

64 Buysse DJ, Reynolds CF, Monk TH, Berman SR, Kupfer DJ: The Pittsburgh Sleep Quality Index: a new instrument for psychiatric practice and research. Psychiatr Res 1989;28:193–213.

65 Thomson J, Oswald I: Effect of oestrogen on the sleep, mood, and anxiety of menopausal women. Br Med J 1977;ii:1317–1319.

66 Schiff I, Regestein Q, Tulchinsky D, Ryan KJ: Effects of estogens on sleep and psychological state of hypogonadal women. JAMA 1979;242:2405–2407.

67 Erlik Y, Tataryn IV, Meldrum DR, Lomax P, Bajorek JG, Judd HL: Association of waking episodes with menopausal hot flushes. JAMA 1981;245:1741–1744.

68 Purdie DW, Empson JAC, Crichton C, MacDonald L: Hormone replacement therapy, sleep quality and psychological wellbeing. Br J Obstet Gynaecol 1995;102:735–739.

69 Scharf MB, McDonald MD, Stover R, Zaretsky N, Berkowitz DV: Effects of estrogen replacement therapy on rates of cyclic alternating patterns and hot-flush events during sleep in postmenopausal women: a pilot study. Clin Ther 1997;19:304–311.

70 Polo-Kantola P, Erkkola R, Helenius H, Irjala K, Polo O: When does estrogen replacement therapy improve sleep quality? Am J Obstet Gynecol 1998; 178:1002–1009.

71 Polo-Kantola P, Erkkola R, Irjala K, Pullinen S, Virtanen I, Polo O: Effect of short-term tranderma estrogen replacement therapy on sleep: a randomized, double-blind crossover trial in postmenopausal women. Fertil Steril 1999;71:873–880.

72 Antonijevis IA, Stalla GK, Steiger A: Modulation of the sleep electroencephalogram by estrogen replacement in postmenopausal women. Am J Obstet Gynecol 2000;182:277–282.

73 Freeman EW, Sammel MD, Lin H, Gracia CR, Kapoor S, Ferdousi T: The role of anxiety and hormonal changes in menopausal hot flashes. Menopause 2005; 12:258–266.

74 Freeman EW, Sammel MD, Lin H, Nelson DB: Associations of hormones and menopausal status with depressed mood in women with no history of depression. Arch Gen Psychiatry 2006;63:375–382.

75 Freeman EW, Sammel MD, Lin H, Gracia CR, Pien GW, Nelson DB, Sheng L: Symptoms associated with menopausal transition and reproductive hormones in midlife women. Obstet Gynecol 2007;110: 230–240.

Robert R. Freedman, PhD
Departments of Psychiatry and Obstetrics and Gynecology, Wayne State University School of Medicine
C.S. Mott Center, 275 E. Hancock
Detroit, MI 48201 (USA)
Fax +1 313–577–8382, E-Mail aa2613@wayne.edu

Soares CN, Warren M (eds): The Menopausal Transition. Interface between Gynecology and Psychiatry.
Key Issues in Mental Health. Basel, Karger, 2009, vol 175, pp 102–114

Managing Depression and Anxiety during the Menopausal Transition and Beyond: The Window of Vulnerability

Benicio N. Frey[a,b] · Claudio N. Soares[a–c]

[a]Women's Health Concerns Clinic, St Joseph's Healthcare Hamilton, Departments of [b]Psychiatry and Behavioural Neurosciences, and [c]Obstetrics and Gynecology, McMaster University, Hamilton, Ont., Canada

Abstract

It has long been recognized that women are at a higher risk than men to develop depression and anxiety and that such increased risk is particularly associated with reproductive cycle events. Moreover, recent prospective studies have demonstrated that the transition to menopause is associated with higher risk for new onset and recurrent depression. A number of biological and environmental factors are independent predictors for depression in this population, including the presence of hot flushes, sleep disturbances, history of severe premenstrual syndrome or postpartum blues, stressful life events, history of depression, socioeconomic status and use of hormones and psychotropic agents. Accumulated evidence suggests that ovarian hormones modulate serotonin and noradrenaline neurotransmission, a process that may be associated with the emergence of depressive symptoms and/or anxiety during periods of hormonal fluctuation in biologically predisposed sub-populations. Transdermal estradiol and serotonergic and noradrenergic antidepressants are efficacious in the treatment of depression and vasomotor symptoms in symptomatic, midlife women. Less is known about tailored treatment strategies for the management of anxiety in this vulnerable population. In this chapter, we reviewed the existing evidence that the menopausal transition may be associated with greater risk for anxiety and depression and the putative underlying mechanisms contributing to this increased risk or 'window of vulnerability'. Hormonal and nonhormonal treatment strategies are critically examined, although more tailored treatment options for this population at risk are scarce. Copyright © 2009 S. Karger AG, Basel

It has long been recognized that women are at higher risk than men to develop depression and such risk is particularly higher during the reproductive years [1]. For instance, while women are 1.7 times as likely as men to develop major depressive disorder (MDD) during their lifetime, this risk has not been observed in childhood years [2] or when most women are predominantly postmenopausal [3]. Similarly, anxiety disorders have been reported to be more prevalent in women as compared to men [4]. Given that gender differences in mood and anxiety disorders seem to emerge after puberty and decline during postmenopausal years, it has been postulated that the fluctuation of gonadal hormones may mediate women's vulnerability to these disturbances. A closer look at women's mood during the reproductive years reveals that about 20–40% of women report moderate-to-severe premenstrual symptoms (PMS) and that 10–12% of postpartum women meet the criteria for postpartum depression (PPD); these two phenomena corroborate the notion that some women are particularly sensitive to develop mood symptoms when facing *normal* changes in the hormonal milieu.

Estrogen receptors are widely distributed throughout the brain [5, 6] and the effects of estrogen have been observed in the hypothalamus, prefrontal cortex, hippocampus and brain stem, cerebral regions known to be closely associated with mood and cognitive regulation [6]. Much of the interaction between estrogen and mood is thought to be associated with the effects of estrogen on monoaminergic neurotransmitters, especially serotonin and norepinephrine [7]. For instance, estrogen regulates serotonin neuronal firing, increases serotonin and norepinephrine synthesis and modulates the availability and gene expression of serotonin and norepinephrine receptors [5, 8]. Notably, selective serotonin and serotonin and norepinephrine reuptake inhibitors (SSRIs and SNRIs) are efficacious in the treatment of hot flashes, the most common symptom of menopausal transition, which is thought to be related to a narrowing of the thermoneutral zone caused by increased noradrenergic tone in the hypothalamus [9]. Taken together, these data suggest that women's brain are constantly challenged to adapt to hormonal variations, which could render some women vulnerable to develop mood and anxiety symptoms when the levels of gonadal hormones are chaotic or unpredictable – such as during the menopausal transition.

The transition to menopause is typically characterized by a complex set of emotional and physical symptoms associated with the progressive decline of ovarian function [10]. Population studies have demonstrated that vasomotor symptoms (hot flashes and night sweats), sleep disturbances and vaginal dryness are particularly higher in peri-/postmenopausal than in premenopausal women [11]. Recently, a number of large-scale, community-based, prospective studies have clearly shown that the menopause transition is a period of heightened risk for recurrent and new-onset depression (as discussed below in detail), which is in line with current hypotheses suggesting that the transition to menopause represents a *window of vulnerability* for depression [12, 13]. Moreover, accumulated evidence shows that hormonal and nonhormonal interventions are useful for the management of affective disorders in perimenopausal women [14, 15]. In this chapter, we review the most relevant studies that investigated the emergence of depressive and anxiety states during the menopausal transition and available evidence-based strategies in the treatment of anxiety and depression in this population.

Epidemiologic Studies

Data from community-based, cross-sectional studies that assessed 'psychological distress' or depression in women during menopausal transition have revealed mixed results [16–18]. In a large multiethnic study of women aged 40–55 years across the United States (n = 10,374), Bromberger et al. [17] found higher scores of psychological distress in early perimenopausal women as compared to pre- and postmenopausal women, after controlling for potential confounders. Another study assessing 1,434 women aged between 45 and 55 years found that depressive symptoms were significantly higher in postmenopausal compared to premenopausal women [16]. On the other hand, Slaven and Lee [19] reported no association between depression and menopausal transition in a community sample of 304 women from Australia, assessed with the Women's Health Questionnaire and the Profile of Mood States scales; the relatively small sample size and the lack of more clear definition of inclusion and exclusion criteria limited the generalization of these findings.

Juang et al. [18] examined a sample of 1,273 women between ages 40 and 54 using the Hospital Anxiety and Depression Scale, and demonstrated that anxiety and depression were significantly associated with the presence of hot flashes in peri and postmenopausal women. Another three studies reported that trait and state anxiety were significantly correlated with the severity of sleep disturbance in women during the menopause transition [20–22]. Importantly, no such association was found in premenopausal women [20], suggesting that the association between anxiety and sleep disturbance may be specific to the menopause transition, possibly due to the higher incidence of hot flashes and night sweats in this period. The association between sleep disruption and anxiety symptoms with the presence of hot flashes found further support in a study that examined users of tamoxifen for breast cancer (n = 113) [23]. Other factors that have been associated with anxiety and depressive symptoms during the menopause transition are: history of stressful live events, history of premenstrual syndrome (PMS) and/or mood disorders, poor social support, lower education, age and live in a rural region [16, 18, 24, 25].

Taken together, some but not all cross-sectional studies suggest that the menopause transition may be associated with a higher risk for depression and anxiety. However, cross-sectional studies are usually unable to examine *temporal changes* in mood and anxiety over the course of the menopausal transition, which can be better evaluated prospectively.

Unlike the cross-sectional studies, most prospective studies [26–30] confirmed the transition to menopause as a period of heightened risk for development of depressive symptoms and/or depression – perhaps with the exception of Kaufert et al. [31]. The Penn Ovarian Aging Study followed 436 women from the community across the menopausal transition for an average of 4 years [28]. In this study, the severity of depressive symptoms, as measured by the Center for Epidemiologic Studies Depression Scale (CES-D) was higher during the transition to menopause and decreased after menopause; these increased risk remained significant after controlling for past history of depression, age, PMS, poor sleep, hot flashes, race and employment status [28]. The authors proposed that depressive and menopause-related symptoms may be mechanistically related, given that history of severe PMS and the presence of hot flashes and sleep disturbance were independent predictors of depressive symptoms and diagnosed MDD. The Massachusetts Women's Health Study is a community-based study that investigated 2,356 middle-aged women for 5 years using the CES-D scale to measure the severity of depressive symptoms across the transition to menopause [26]. Perimenopausal women exhibited an increased risk for depression and such risk was even higher among those with menopause-related symptoms, such as hot flashes and night sweats. Two other independent community-based studies evaluated large samples of middle-aged women, the Study of Women's Health Across the Nation (n = 3,302) [27] and the Seattle Midlife Women's Health Study (n = 508) [30]; both studies also revealed a heightened risk for depression during the perimenopausal period, with the presence of hot flashes being an independent risk factor.

In order to assess whether the transition to menopause increases the risk for *new-onset* depression, two long-term prospective studies followed women with no history of depression across the menopause transition [32, 33]. In the Harvard Study of Moods and Cycles, 460 never-depressed women were followed-up for 6–8 years and those who entered the perimenopause were nearly twice as likely (OR = 1.8 [1.0–3.2]) to develop significant depressive symptoms compared to those who remained premenopausal. In this study, the presence of vasomotor symptoms and history of significant life events were independent predictors of higher risk for depression [32]. In the Penn Ovarian Aging Study, 231 women with no history of depression were followed for 8 years; perimenopausal women were 4 times more likely to have high CES-D scores and twice as likely to meet criteria for MDD than premenopausal women [33]. In addition, greater variation of estradiol and FSH levels (as calculated from the standard deviation of hormonal levels) was associated with both higher depressive scores and diagnosed MDD, which suggests that fluctuations of hormonal levels, rather than their absolute levels, may play a significant role as a trigger for depressive symptoms in biologically vulnerable women. This is consistent with previous studies reporting that hormone fluctuations, rather than absolute hormonal levels, are more likely to be associated with the onset of depressive symptoms during certain female reproductive life events [30, 34]. Several other factors have also been associated with depression during menopausal transition, including age, ethnicity (higher risk in African-American, lower risk in Asian populations), education, family history of depression, postpartum blues or depression, body mass index, use of hormone therapy or antidepressants, cigarette smoking and stressful life events [26–30] reinforcing the complex, multi-faceted aspect of depression.

Rocca et al. [35] conducted a cohort study of women who underwent oophorectomy before the onset of menopause (average follow-up 25 years) and matched these subjects by age with subjects from the same community who had not undergone an oophorectomy. Those who underwent surgery (bilateral oophorectomy, n = 666) had a significant increased risk for developing depressive symptoms (HR = 1.54, 95% CI = 1.04–2.26) and anxiety symptoms (HR = 2.29, 95% CI = 1.33–3.95) when compared to the referent group (n = 673). These results remained significant after adjusting for age, education, and type of surgery; more over, the risks for even greater among those who underwent surgery at younger age [35]. The authors speculate possible mechanisms to explain the association between estrogen deficiency caused by oophorectomy prior to the onset of menopause and the occurrence of symptoms of anxiety and depression: the loss of neuro-protective effects attributed to normal estrogen levels throughout the reproductive life years; the resulting deficiency of testosterone and progesterone after surgery and its impact on the HPG axis; putative genetic variants that increase the risk for these outcomes (ovarian disorders and psychiatric disturbances) independently.

Longitudinal studies looking specifically at risk for anxiety in perimenopausal women have that natural (i.e. nonsurgical) transition to menopause is associated with increased risk for anxiety, after controlling for the presence or severity of depression. Freeman et al. [36] followed-up 436 midlife women for 6 years and found that hot flashes were strongly associated with anxiety, especially in women who were in the early menopausal transition. There was a 'dose-response' effect between the severity of anxiety and the presence of hot flashes, with women with high anxiety scores being 4 times more likely to report hot flashes as compared to women with no anxiety; those with moderate anxiety scores had a 3-fold increased risk for hot flashes. Anxiety remained strongly associated with hot flashes after controlling for important factors, such as depression, age, race, menopause stage, body mass index, smoking and estradiol levels. More recently, the same group investigated the relationship between menopausal stage and anxiety, depression, mood swings, headache and concentration difficulties in the same cohort after 9 years of follow-up [37]. Anxiety appeared to achieve its peak during the early menopausal transition and returned to premenopausal levels after menopause. In addition, women with a history of premenstrual syndrome were twice as likely to report anxiety compared to those with no history of premenstrual syndrome. In the SWAN study, the association between vasomotor symptoms and a number of health and lifestyle factors was examined in 3,198 midlife women during a 6-year follow-up [38]. Interestingly, this study suggested a mutual relationship between anxiety and vasomotor symptoms – at baseline, women reporting more vasomotor symptoms were more likely to be anxious than women with fewer vasomotor symptoms (53.6 vs. 19.1%; p < 0.0001). Conversely, more baseline anxiety was an independent factor for more vasomotor symptoms at the end of the 6-year follow-up (OR = 3.10; CI = 2.33–4.12) [38]. In summary, long-term, community-based longitudinal studies provide strong evidence that the menopausal transition is a period of higher risk for depression and anxiety. While multiple risk factors appear to independently modulate such a risk, the presence of vasomotor symptoms and hormonal fluctuation seem to be closely associated with emotional disturbance.

Thus, it is likely that treatment strategies to ameliorate menopause-related symptoms can not only improve women's quality of life, but also may decrease the likelihood of emotional disturbance in this population at risk.

Treatment Strategies

Treatment strategies specifically targeting the management of depression and anxiety during menopausal transition are scarce. The few randomized, placebo-controlled trials (RCTs) conducted to date have primarily focused on the efficacy of hormone therapies in depressed women. While a number of open trials are suggestive that selective serotonin and serotonin-norepinephrine reuptake inhibitors (SSRIs and SNRIs) are effective in the treatment of depression in perimenopausal women, large RCTs are lacking. In addition, the vast majority of treatment studies assessed anxiety symptoms as secondary outcomes or included populations with low anxiety levels. Nevertheless, as further discussed, available evidence suggest that both hormonal and nonhormonal agents are useful tools for the management of depression and anxiety in perimenopausal women.

Depression

The few RCTs that investigated the antidepressant effects of estrogen found that transdermal 17β-estradiol 50–100 μg when used for 6–12 weeks is efficacious for the treatment of depression (major depression minor depression or dysthymia) in perimenopausal women, with remission rates of 68–80% as compared to 20–22% with placebo [14, 15]. Notably, 100 μg transdermal estradiol for 8 weeks was not effective in the treatment of depression in postmenopausal women [39]. These studies provide strong evidence suggesting that the transition to menopause might not only be a critical period of higher risk for depression, but also a *window of opportunity* for the use of hormonal strategies in the management of depression [12].

The initial findings from the Women's Health Initiative (WHI) had a significant, negative impact on the physicians' and patients' perception of the long-term safety and benefits of hormone replacement therapies (HRT) [40; [more details in the chapter by Warren et al., this volume]; as a result, many health professional and their patients became more cautious or reluctant to initiate HRT or to stay on HRT for longer periods of time; others started seeking nonhormonal strategies to improve menopause-related physical and psychological discomforts [41, 42]. In Ontario, Canada, for example, there was a sharp decrease in prescriptions of HRT that occurred in parallel with a marked increase in prescriptions of antidepressants to women 40 years of age or older [43]. Several open trials have provided evidence that serotonergic and noradrenergic agents are efficacious for the management of depression [44, 45] and vasomotor symptoms [46–48] in perimenopausal and/or postmenopausal women. Remission rates of depressive symptoms were observed in 86.6 and 75% of depressed women after monotherapy with citalopram and escitalopram, respectively [45, 49]. In these studies, there was a significant improvement in menopause-related symptoms (e.g. hot flashes, night sweats, somatic complaints). Mirtazapine and citalopram were tested as adjunctive treatments to estrogen therapy in depressed peri-/postmenopausal women, with remission rates of 87.5% with mirtazapine and 91.6% with citalopram [45, 50]. Interestingly, a pooled analysis of eight RCT studies found that women >50 years achieved higher remission rates with the SNRI venlafaxine (48%) as compared to SSRIs (28%) while not receiving estrogen therapies (ET), whereas the difference between the two treatment groups was significantly reduced among those receiving ET [51]. Based on these intriguing results, one could speculate that postmenopausal women might benefit from the priming/synergistic effect of ET while on SSRIs; in the absence of ET, postmenopausal women would have a more robust response to antidepressants that act preferably on noradrenergic neurotransmission. Although intriguing, this hypothesis warrants further investigation in larger, prospective RCTs and should not discourage physicians or patients to use SSRIs to manage MDD during postmenopausal years. A recent study investigated the use of the SNRI duloxetine in the treatment of depression in postmenopausal women and found remission rates of 78.6% after 8 weeks [44]. Importantly, duloxetine showed a positive effect in the amelioration of menopause-related symptoms as well.

Botanical agents have been investigated as nonhormonal alternatives for the treatment of menopause-associated symptoms, with only limited evidence suggesting that these agents reduce the frequency and severity of vasomotor symptoms. Two small RCTs suggested that Black Cohosh (Actaea racemosa) is more effective than placebo in the treatment of mild-to-moderate vasomotor symptoms [52, 53]. In a recent meta-analysis including 43 RCTs, soy isoflavone extracts showed a small positive effect over placebo, which is observed after 12 weeks of treatment [54]. Newton et al. [55] tested the efficacy of 3 herbal regimens and hormone therapy for relief of vasomotor symptoms compared with placebo in a 1-year randomized, double-blind, placebo-controlled trial (n = 353). Treatment groups included Black Cohosh alone (160 mg/day), multibotanical with Black Cohosh (200 mg) and 9 other ingredients, multibotanical plus dietary soy counseling and conjugated equine estrogen, 0.625 mg (with or without medroxyprogesterone acetate), or placebo. At 12 months, symptom intensity was significantly worse with the multibotanical plus soy intervention than with placebo. Moreover, the difference in vasomotor symptoms between placebo and any of the herbal treatments at any time point of the study was minimal – less than 1 symptom per day.

To date, no studies have investigated the efficacy of botanical agents in the treatment of peri-/postmenopausal women with a major depressive episode. Nonetheless, one RCT that investigated 301 women with climacteric complaints showed a 41.8% improvement in Hamilton Depression Rating Scale (HAM-D) scores from baseline

(18.9 ± 2.2) to 16 weeks (11.0 ± 3.8) with a combination of Black Cohosh and St. John's Wort (*Hypericum perforatum*) [56]. These results are consistent with those from a 12-week open-trial with St. John's Wort in 111 women (aged between 43 and 65 years) with climacteric symptoms, in which participants showed significant improvement of psychological and psychosomatic symptoms [57]. Taken together, available evidence indicate that transdermal estrogen, SSRIs and SNRIs are effective in the treatment of depression during the menopausal transition. More systematic data on botanical agents and other nonhormonal treatment strategies for depression in peri-/post-menopausal women are lacking, but women with lifetime history of depression may benefit from the mild effects of such agents on menopause-related symptoms – after all, the presence of vasomotor symptoms and other menopause-related complaints appears to be associated with a higher risk for depression during menopausal transition [27, 30].

Anxiety

To date, no studies have investigated the effects of hormonal therapies for the treatment of anxiety in peri-/postmenopausal women. Some studies have assessed the impact of hormone therapies on symptoms of anxiety as a secondary outcome measure. For instance, a study that evaluated 70 women with climacteric symptoms observed that those who opted for receiving HRT (n = 35) reported lower anxiety, sleep and somatic complaints than women who chose not to receive HRT (n = 35) [58]. Three RCTs that assessed secondary effects of HRT on anxiety symptoms in peri- and postmeno-pausal women reported little or no effects [59–61]. A large trial that randomized 419 postmenopausal women to 4 different HRT regimens found only modest effects of hormone treatments on anxiety scores after up to 9 years of follow-up [62]. However, it is important to highlight that these negative findings may be explained in part by a 'floor effect', since most study participants revealed relatively low anxiety scores at study entry. Two studies investigated the effects of tibolone, a selective estrogen recep-tor modulator (SERM), on symptoms of anxiety and depression. One study that com-pared 19 postmenopausal women using tibolone for 6 months with 25 women not on any medications found that tibolone had a positive effect in decreasing anxiety scores [63]. However, Hamilton Anxiety Rating Scale (HAMA) scores decreased from 7.8 ± 7.7 at baseline to 5.5 ± 4.3 at 6 months, which may not have been clinically significant. In a RCT, 75 women who had hysterectomy-oophorectomy for benign conditions were randomized to tibolone, transdermal estradiol or placebo and followed-up for 6 months. Improvement in anxiety and depression scores was observed with both active treatments compared to placebo, while no differences between tibolone and transdermal estradiol were documented [64]. Again, the relatively low baseline anxi-ety scores (HAMA scores ~9–10) limit the generalization of the results. Studies with well-defined population presenting with high anxiety scores are necessary to better investigate the potential use of hormone therapies in the treatment of anxiety in women during the menopause transition.

Similarly, no studies to date have addressed the effects of antidepressants for the management of anxiety disorders in peri-/postmenopausal women and available data derived from studies of either healthy or depressed subpopulations. Nonetheless, existing evidence suggest that antidepressants may have a positive effect in alleviating anxiety symptoms among midlife/postmenopausal women. Two open trials observed a modest anxiolytic effect with trazodone and paroxetine for the management of menopausal symptoms in otherwise healthy peri-/postmenopausal women [65, 66]. Three open trials evaluated the effects of citalopram, venlafaxine and duloxetine in peri-/postmenopausal women with major depression and reported reduction in anxiety scores as secondary outcome measures [44, 45, 67]. In all these studies, beneficial effects on both depressive and anxiety scores were observed after 8 weeks of therapy. Importantly, these antidepressants had also a positive effect in alleviating menopause-related symptoms, such as hot flashes and night sweats. Consistently, a larger study of perimenopausal women with depression reported a significant improvement in depression, anxiety and menopause scores after 3 months of treatment with fluvoxamine (n = 53) or paroxetine (n = 52) [68]. Although results with antidepressants are encouraging, future studies examining the efficacy of antidepressants in women with primary anxiety disorders in the context of menopause transition are warranted.

A number of studies investigated the use of botanical agents in the management of anxiety symptoms in peri-/postmenopausal women. One open trial assessed the effects of St. John's Wort in 111 women between 43 and 65 years of age and found that 79% of women reported improvement in climacteric complains [57]. In one RCT, 149 individuals (67% women) with a primary diagnosis of somatoform disorder were allocated to St. John's Wort or placebo and the HAM-A total score was used as the primary outcome measure [69]. In this study, a significant decrease in total HAM-A scores was observed after 42 days of treatment with St. John's Wort. Two small RCTs evaluated the effects of Kava extract on anxiety symptoms in perimenopausal [70] and postmenopausal women [71]; the efficacy of Kava extract plus calcium supplementation in reducing anxiety symptoms was superior than calcium supplementation only ('control group') [70]. The combination of Kava extracts + HT was more efficacious than HT alone to alleviate anxiety symptoms in 40 postmenopausal women and this effect was maintained after 6 months of treatment [71]. Although preliminary, these findings suggest that Kava extract may be a useful option in the management of anxiety during menopausal transition and postmenopausal years. However, clinicians should be aware of the potential hepatotoxicity of Kava extract as well as its various drug-drug interactions [72]. A small open-trial tested the efficacy of Korean red ginseng on anxiety scores in 12 postmenopausal women with menopausal symptoms and found a small effect of this compound for the reduction of anxiety symptoms after one month of treatment [73]. Negative effects of *Ginko biloba* and *Panax ginseng* (Gincosan) on anxiety, mood and menopausal symptoms were reported in a RCT

involving 70 postmenopausal women [74]. More recently, 64 peri- and postmenopausal women were randomly allocated to either Black Cohosh or transdermal estradiol and both treatments were equally effective in decreasing anxiety, depressive and
vasomotor symptoms [75]. Lastly, negative effects of isoflavones and Valerian extract
were reported by two RCTs [76, 77]. In summary, studies investigating the effects
of botanical agents in the management of anxiety in peri/postmenopausal women
are limited, given that anxiety was a secondary outcome measure in most studies.
Therefore, RCTs assessing peri- and postmenopausal women with well-defined, anxiety disorders as primary diagnoses are necessary.

Conclusions

Despite robust evidence (epidemiologic studies, RCTs) that the menopausal transition may constitute a window of vulnerability for the development of mood and anxiety disorders, little is known about the underlying mechanisms that contribute to
the occurrence of this phenomenon. Moreover, more tailored treatment strategies to
address the spectrum of physical and psychological complaints at this stage in life are
lacking. In the post-WHI era, it is imperative that health professionals become aware
of the putative impact of menopause (natural or surgical) on psychological well being,
particularly among those who are unable or unwilling to use hormone therapies.
More research on non-hormonal options (i.e. selective estrogen receptor modulators
(SERMs), herbal supplements, psychotropic agents) should be strongly encouraged to
expand the portfolio of treatment strategies available for this population at risk.

References

1 Kessler RC, McGonagle KA, Swartz M, Blazer DG, Nelson CB: Sex and depression in the National Comorbidity Survey. I. Lifetime prevalence, chronicity and recurrence. J Affect Disord 1993;29:85–96.

2 Birmaher B, Ryan ND, Williamson DE, Brent DA, Kaufman J, Dahl RE, Perel J, Nelson B: Childhood and adolescent depression: a review of the past 10 years. Part I. J Am Acad Child Adolesc Psychiatry 1996;35:1427–1439.

3 Bebbington P, Dunn G, Jenkins R, Lewis G, Brugha T, Farrell M, Meltzer H: The influence of age and sex on the prevalence of depressive conditions: report from the National Survey of Psychiatric Morbidity. Int Rev Psychiatry 2003;15:74–83.

4 Kessler RC, McGonagle KA, Zhao S, Nelson CB, Hughes M, Eshleman S, Wittchen HU, Kendler KS: Lifetime and 12-month prevalence of DSM-III-R psychiatric disorders in the United States: results from the National Comorbidity Survey. Arch Gen Psychiatry 1994;51:8–19.

5 McEwen BS: Estrogens effects on the brain: multiple sites and molecular mechanisms (invited review). J Appl Physiol 2001;91:2785–2801.

6 Morrison JH, Brinton RD, Schmidt PJ, Gore AC: Estrogen, menopause, and the aging brain: how basic neuroscience can inform hormone therapy in women. J Neurosci 2006;26:10332–10348.

7 McEwen BS, Alves SE: Estrogen actions in the central nervous system. Endocr Rev 1999;20:279–307.

8 Deecher D, Andree TH, Sloan D, Schechter LE: From menarche to menopause: exploring the underlying biology of depression in women experiencing hormonal changes. Psychoneuroendocrinology 2008; 33:3–17.

9 Freedman RR: Pathophysiology and treatment of menopausal hot flashes. Semin Reprod Med 2005;23:117–125.

10 Santoro N: The menopausal transition. Am J Med 2005;118(suppl 12B):8–13.

11 Montgomery JC, Studd JW: Psychological and sexual aspects of the menopause. Br J Hosp Med 1991; 45:300–302.

12 Soares CN: Depression during the menopausal transition: window of vulnerability or continuum of risk? Menopause 2008;15:207–209.

13 Soares CN, Zitek B: Reproductive hormone sensitivity and risk for depression across the female life cycle: a continuum of vulnerability? J Psychiatry Neurosci 2008;33:331–343.

14 Soares CN, Almeida OP, Joffe H, Cohen LS: Efficacy of estradiol for the treatment of depressive disorders in perimenopausal women: a double-blind, randomized, placebo-controlled trial. Arch Gen Psychiatry 2001;58:529–534.

15 Schmidt PJ, Nieman L, Danaceau MA, Tobin MB, Roca CA, Murphy JH, Rubinow DR: Estrogen replacement in perimenopause-related depression: a preliminary report. Am J Obstet Gynecol 2000; 183:414–420.

16 Amore M, Di Donato P, Berti A, Palareti A, Chirico C, Papalini A, Zucchini S: Sexual and psychological symptoms in the climacteric years. Maturitas 2007; 56:303–311.

17 Bromberger JT, Meyer PM, Kravitz HM, Sommer B, Cordal A, Powell L, Ganz PA, Sutton-Tyrrell K: Psychologic distress and natural menopause: a multiethnic community study. Am J Publ Health 2001; 91:1435–1442.

18 Juang KD, Wang SJ, Lu SR, Lee SJ, Fuh JL: Hot flashes are associated with psychological symptoms of anxiety and depression in peri- and post- but not premenopausal women. Maturitas 2005;52:119–126.

19 Slaven L, Lee C: Mood and symptom reporting among middle-aged women: the relationship between menopausal status, hormone replacement therapy, and exercise participation. Health Psychol 1997;16:203–208.

20 Baker A, Simpson S, Dawson D: Sleep disruption and mood changes associated with menopause. J Psychosom Res 1997;43:359–369.

21 Kloss JD, Tweedy K, Gilrain K: Psychological factors associated with sleep disturbance among perimenopausal women. Behav Sleep Med 2004;2: 177–190.

22 Thurston RC, Blumenthal JA, Babyak MA, Sherwood A: Association between hot flashes, sleep complaints, and psychological functioning among healthy menopausal women. Int J Behav Med 2006;13:163–172.

23 Hunter MS, Grunfeld EA, Mittal S, Sikka P, Ramirez AJ, Fentiman I, Hamed H: Menopausal symptoms in women with breast cancer: prevalence and treatment preferences. Psychooncology 2004;13:769–778.

24 Binfa L, Castelo-Branco C, Blumel JE, Cancelo MJ, Bonilla H, Munoz I, Vergara V, Izaguirre H, Sarra S, Rios RV: Influence of psycho-social factors on climacteric symptoms. Maturitas 2004;48:425–431.

25 Malacara JM, Canto de Cetina T, Bassol S, Gonzalez N, Cacique L, Vera-Ramirez ML, Nava LE: Symptoms at pre- and postmenopause in rural and urban women from three States of Mexico. Maturitas 2002;43:11–19.

26 Avis NE, Brambilla D, McKinlay SM, Vass K: A longitudinal analysis of the association between menopause and depression. Results from the Massachusetts Women's Health Study. Ann Epidemiol 1994;4:214–220.

27 Bromberger JT, Matthews KA, Schott LL, Brockwell S, Avis NE, Kravitz HM, Everson-Rose SA, Gold EB, Sowers M, Randolph JF Jr: Depressive symptoms during the menopausal transition: The Study of Women's Health Across the Nation (SWAN). J Affect Disord 2007.

28 Freeman EW, Sammel MD, Liu L, Gracia CR, Nelson DB, Hollander L: Hormones and menopausal status as predictors of depression in women in transition to menopause. Arch Gen Psychiatry 2004;61:62–70.

29 Maartens LW, Knottnerus JA, Pop VJ: Menopausal transition and increased depressive symptomatology: a community based prospective study. Maturitas 2002;42:195–200.

30 Woods NF, Smith-DiJulio K, Percival DB, Tao EY, Mariella A, Mitchell S: Depressed mood during the menopausal transition and early postmenopause: observations from the Seattle Midlife Women's Health Study. Menopause 2008;15:223–232.

31 Kaufert PA, Gilbert P, Tate R: The Manitoba Project: a re-examination of the link between menopause and depression. Maturitas 1992;14:143–155.

32 Cohen LS, Soares CN, Vitonis AF, Otto MW, Harlow BL: Risk for new onset of depression during the menopausal transition: The Harvard Study of Moods and Cycles. Arch Gen Psychiatry 2006;63: 385–390.

33 Freeman EW, Sammel MD, Lin H, Nelson DB: Associations of hormones and menopausal status with depressed mood in women with no history of depression. Arch Gen Psychiatry 2006;63:375–382.

34 Bloch M, Schmidt PJ, Danaceau M, Murphy J, Nieman L, Rubinow DR: Effects of gonadal steroids in women with a history of postpartum depression. Am J Psychiatry 2000;157:924–930.

35 Rocca WA, Grossardt BR, Geda YE, Gostout BS, Bower JH, Maraganore DM, de Andrade M, Melton LJ 3rd: Long-term risk of depressive and anxiety symptoms after early bilateral oophorectomy. Menopause 2008;15:1050–1059.

36 Freeman EW, Sammel MD, Lin H, Gracia CR, Kapoor S, Ferdousi T: The role of anxiety and hormonal changes in menopausal hot flashes. Menopause 2005;12:258–266.

37 Freeman EW, Sammel MD, Lin H, Gracia CR, Kapoor S: Symptoms in the menopausal transition: hormone and behavioral correlates. Obstet Gynecol 2008;111:127–136.

38 Gold EB, Colvin A, Avis N, Bromberger J, Greendale GA, Powell L, Sternfeld B, Matthews K: Longitudinal analysis of the association between vasomotor symptoms and race/ethnicity across the menopausal transition: study of women's health across the nation. Am J Public Health 2006;96:1226–1235.

39 Morrison MF, Kallan MJ, Ten Have T, Katz I, Tweedy K, Battistini M: Lack of efficacy of estradiol for depression in postmenopausal women: a randomized, controlled trial. Biol Psychiatry 2004;55:406–412.

40 Rossouw JE, Anderson GL, Prentice RL, LaCroix AZ, Kooperberg C, Stefanick ML, Jackson RD, Beresford SA, Howard BV, Johnson KC, Kotchen JM, Ockene J: Risks and benefits of estrogen plus progestin in healthy postmenopausal women: principal results From the Women's Health Initiative randomized controlled trial. JAMA 2002;288:321–333.

41 Hackley B, Rousseau ME: CEU: managing menopausal symptoms after the women's health initiative. J Midwifery Womens Health 2004;49:87–95.

42 Kessel B, Kronenberg F: The role of complementary and alternative medicine in management of menopausal symptoms. Endocrinol Metab Clin North Am 2004;33:717–739.

43 McIntyre RS, Konarski JZ, Grigoriadis S, Fan NC, Mancini DA, Fulton KA, Stewart DE, Kennedy SH: Hormone replacement therapy and antidepressant prescription patterns: a reciprocal relationship. CMA J 2005;172:57–59.

44 Joffe H, Soares CN, Petrillo LF, Viguera AC, Somley BL, Koch JK, Cohen LS: Treatment of depression and menopause-related symptoms with the serotonin-norepinephrine reuptake inhibitor duloxetine. J Clin Psychiatry 2007;68:943–950.

45 Soares CN, Poitras JR, Prouty J, Alexander AB, Shifren JL, Cohen LS: Efficacy of citalopram as a monotherapy or as an adjunctive treatment to estrogen therapy for perimenopausal and postmenopausal women with depression and vasomotor symptoms. J Clin Psychiatry 2003;64:473–479.

46 Evans ML, Pritts E, Vittinghoff E, McClish K, Morgan KS, Jaffe RB: Management of postmenopausal hot flushes with venlafaxine hydrochloride: a randomized, controlled trial. Obstet Gynecol 2005;105:161–166.

47 Speroff L, Gass M, Constantine G, Olivier S: Efficacy and tolerability of desvenlafaxine succinate treatment for menopausal vasomotor symptoms: a randomized controlled trial. Obstet Gynecol 2008; 111:77–87.

48 Stearns V, Beebe KL, Iyengar M, Dube E: Paroxetine controlled release in the treatment of menopausal hot flashes: a randomized controlled trial. JAMA 2003;289:2827–2834.

49 Soares CN, Arsenio H, Joffe H, Bankier B, Cassano P, Petrillo LF, Cohen LS: Escitalopram versus ethinyl estradiol and norethindrone acetate for symptomatic peri- and postmenopausal women: impact on depression, vasomotor symptoms, sleep, and quality of life. Menopause 2006;13:780–786.

50 Joffe H, Groninger H, Soares CN, Nonacs R, Cohen LS: An open trial of mirtazapine in menopausal women with depression unresponsive to estrogen replacement therapy. J Womens Health Gend Based Med 2001;10:999–1004.

51 Thase ME, Entsuah R, Cantillon M, Kornstein SG: Relative antidepressant efficacy of venlafaxine and SSRIs: sex-age interactions. J Womens Health (Larchmt) 2005;14:609–616.

52 Osmers R, Friede M, Liske E, Schnitker J, Freudenstein J, Henneicke-von Zepelin HH: Efficacy and safety of isopropanolic Black Cohosh extract for climacteric symptoms. Obstet Gynecol 2005;105(5 Pt 1):1074–1083.

53 Wuttke W, Jarry H, Christoffel V, Spengler B, Seidlova-Wuttke D: Chaste tree (*Vitex agnus castus*): pharmacology and clinical indications. Phytomedicine 2003;10:348–357.

54 Nelson HD, Vesco KK, Haney E, Fu R, Nedrow A, Miller J, Nicolaidis C, Walker M, Humphrey L: Nonhormonal therapies for menopausal hot flashes: systematic review and meta-analysis. JAMA 2006; 295:2057–2071.

55 Newton KM, Reed SD, LaCroix AZ, Grothaus LC, Ehrlich K, Guiltinan J: Treatment of vasomotor symptoms of menopause with Black Cohosh, multibotanicals, soy, hormone therapy, or placebo: a randomized trial. Ann Intern Med 2006;145:869–879.

56 Uebelhack R, Blohmer JU, Graubaum HJ, Busch R, Gruenwald J, Wernecke KD: Black cohosh and St. John's Wort for climacteric complaints: a randomized trial. Obstet Gynecol 2006;107:247–255.

57 Grube B, Walper A, Wheatley D: St. John's Wort extract: efficacy for menopausal symptoms of psychological origin. Adv Ther 1999;16:177–186.

58 Boyle GJ, Murrihy R: A preliminary study of hormone replacement therapy and psychological mood states in perimenopausal women. Psychol Rep 2001;88:160–170.

59 Gambacciani M, Ciaponi M, Cappagli B, Monteleone P, Benussi C, Bevilacqua G, Genazzani AR: Effects of low-dose, continuous combined estradiol and noretisterone acetate on menopausal quality of life in early postmenopausal women. Maturitas 2003;44: 157–163.

60 Haines CJ, Yim SF, Chung TK, Lam CW, Lau EW, Ng MH, Chin R, Lee DT: A prospective, randomized, placebo-controlled study of the dose effect of oral oestradiol on menopausal symptoms, psychological well being, and quality of life in postmenopausal Chinese women. Maturitas 2003;44:207–214.

61 Khoo SK, Coglan M, Battistutta D, Tippett V, Raphael B: Hormonal treatment and psychological function during the menopausal transition: an evaluation of the effects of conjugated estrogens/cyclic medroxyprogesterone acetate. Climacteric 1998;1: 55–62.

62 Heikkinen J, Vaheri R, Timonen U: A 10-year follow-up of postmenopausal women on long-term continuous combined hormone replacement therapy: update of safety and quality-of-life findings. J Br Menopause Soc 2006;12:115–125.

63 Gulseren L, Kalafat D, Mandaci H, Gulseren S, Camli L: Effects of tibolone on the quality of life, anxiety-depression levels and cognitive functions in natural menopause: an observational follow-up study. Aust NZ J Obstet Gynaecol 2005;45:71–73.

64 Baksu A, Ayas B, Citak S, Kalan A, Baksu B, Goker N: Efficacy of tibolone and transdermal estrogen therapy on psychological symptoms in women following surgical menopause. Int J Gynaecol Obstet 2005;91:58–62.

65 Pansini F, Albertazzi P, Bonaccorsi G, Zanotti L, Porto S, Dossi L, Campobasso C, Mollica G: Trazodone: a non-hormonal alternative for neurovegetative climacteric symptoms. Clin Exp Obstet Gynecol 1995;22:341–344.

66 Stearns V, Isaacs C, Rowland J, Crawford J, Ellis MJ, Kramer R, Lawrence W, Hanfelt JJ, Hayes DF: A pilot trial assessing the efficacy of paroxetine hydrochloride (Paxil) in controlling hot flashes in breast cancer survivors. Ann Oncol 2000;11:17–22.

67 Ladd CO, Newport DJ, Ragan KA, Loughhead A, Stowe ZN: Venlafaxine in the treatment of depressive and vasomotor symptoms in women with perimenopausal depression. Depress Anxiety 2005;22: 94–97.

68 Ushiroyama T, Ikeda A, Ueki M: Evaluation of double-blind comparison of fluvoxamine and paroxetine in the treatment of depressed outpatients in menopause transition. J Med 2004;35:151–162.

69 Volz HP, Murck H, Kasper S, Moller HJ: St John's Wort extract (LI 160) in somatoform disorders: results of a placebo-controlled trial. Psychopharmacology (Berl) 2002;164:294–300.

70 Cagnacci A, Arangino S, Renzi A, Zanni AL, Malmusi S, Volpe A: Kava-Kava administration reduces anxiety in perimenopausal women. Maturitas 2003;44: 103–109.

71 De Leo V, la Marca A, Morgante G, Lanzetta D, Florio P, Petraglia F: Evaluation of combining kava extract with hormone replacement therapy in the treatment of postmenopausal anxiety. Maturitas 2001;39:185–188.

72 Geller SE, Studee L: Botanical and dietary supplements for mood and anxiety in menopausal women. Menopause 2007;14:541–549.

73 Tode T, Kikuchi Y, Hirata J, Kita T, Nakata H, Nagata I: Effect of Korean red ginseng on psychological functions in patients with severe climacteric syndromes. Int J Gynaecol Obstet 1999;67:169–174.

74 Hartley DE, Elsabagh S, File SE: Gincosan (a combination of *Ginkgo biloba* and *Panax ginseng*): the effects on mood and cognition of 6 and 12 weeks' treatment in post-menopausal women. Nutr Neurosci 2004;7:325–333.

75 Nappi RE, Malavasi B, Brundu B, Facchinetti F: Efficacy of *Cimicifuga racemosa* on climacteric complaints: a randomized study versus low-dose transdermal estradiol. Gynecol Endocrinol 2005;20: 30–35.

76 Andreatini R, Sartori VA, Seabra ML, Leite JR: Effect of valepotriates (valerian extract) in generalized anxiety disorder: a randomized placebo-controlled pilot study. Phytother Res 2002;16:650–654.

77 Casini ML, Marelli G, Papaleo E, Ferrari A, D'Ambrosio F, Unfer V: Psychological assessment of the effects of treatment with phytoestrogens on postmenopausal women: a randomized, double-blind, crossover, placebo-controlled study. Fertil Steril 2006; 85:972–978.

Claudio N. Soares, MD, PhD, FRCPC
Academic Head, Mood Disorders Division; Director, WHCC
301 James St South, FB 638
Hamilton, Ont. L8P 3B6 (Canada)
Tel. +1 905 522 1155, Ext. 33605, Fax +1 905 521 6098, E-Mail csoares@mcmaster.ca

Soares CN, Warren M (eds): The Menopausal Transition. Interface between Gynecology and Psychiatry.
Key Issues in Mental Health. Basel, Karger, 2009, vol 175, pp 115–126

Psychotic Disorders and Menopause: The Untold Story

Anita Riecher-Rössler

Psychiatric Outpatient Department, University Hospital Basel, Basel, Switzerland

Abstract

This chapter aims to give an overview on the influence of menopause on psychotic disorders. Menopause is associated with a loss of estrogens; estrogen has important neuro- and psychoprotective activities, thus its decline and/or instability may trigger or aggravate mental disorders including psychotic ones. As a result, perimenopause may lead to an enhanced risk of first onset of schizophrenic psychoses or 'late-onset schizophrenia'. Women with pre-existing chronic schizophrenia tend to have a deterioration of their illness after menopause and a higher demand for antipsychotic medication. Apart from the psychotic symptoms, many other conditions can be aggravated by the loss of estrogens, including sleep disturbances, irritability, depression, cognitive impairment and sexual problems. In addition, many females with diagnosis of schizophrenia may present with premature menopause due to antipsychotic or stress-induced hyperprolactinamia and the subsequent gonadal suppression. Apart from psychotherapy and social measures, replacement of 17β-estradiol may be helpful in women with schizophrenia in the perimenopause and early postmenopause, but its use might also carry some risks. More research is needed on the indications and contraindications for hormone replacement in this context.

Approximately 100 years ago, the age of menopause in our society often exceeded women's life expectancy, with the result that many women did not experience the medical problems nowadays associated with the menopause. Today the average life expectancy of a female in our society exceeds 80 years and, consequently, women now live more than one third of their lives during the postmenopause.

In addition to the obvious physical changes occurring around the menopause, this phase of life is often burdened with numerous emotional stressors that have already been explored in other chapters of this book.

The sudden loss of estrogen activity may also have a negative impact on mental functioning. There is an increasing body of evidence from basic science, epidemiological data and interventional studies to indicate that estrogens play a role in positively influencing mental well-being [1, 2, for review]. From the clinical point of view, depressive symptoms and even an upsurge in the incidence of some severe mental disorders, such as schizophrenia [3], have been observed around the menopause, suggesting direct involvement of the estrogen activity.

Methodological Problems

Research on the relationship between menopause and mental health shows some difficulties and methodological limitations, which are briefly described here.

First, 'menopause' is often not clearly defined and not well differentiated from 'perimenopause' and 'postmenopause', even menopause is sometimes not differentiated from natural surgical menopause. Furthermore, many studies have relied on self-reporting of women and did not include measurements of hormonal serum levels. Fourth, studies were quite often based on clinical samples rather than community-based cohorts. Fifth, many studies have only examined the occurrence of mental disorders cross-sectionally and not through longitudinal assessment of well-established cohorts.

Finally, the extent to which the menopause itself affects psychological symptoms is of difficult interpretation, particularly given the fact that the normal aging and the menopausal transition share common biological and psychosocial characteristics.

Role of Estrogens in Schizophrenic Psychoses

Estrogens: A Protective Factor in Schizophrenia?

Historical Findings
Since the last century, psychiatrists have been able to recognize the possible association between schizophrenia and estrogens (for review, see [4]). On the one hand, early clinicians such as Kraepelin and Kretschmer described signs of *chronic* 'hypo-estrogenism' in women with schizophrenia. On the other hand, there have been observations on the association between estrogen levels and *acute* psychotic symptomatology. Kraft-Ebing was among the first to describe women becoming psychotic before or during menstruation, i.e. when estrogen levels are relatively low. Kraepelin even created a separate diagnostic category, labelled 'menstrual psychosis'. Kretschmer reported cases where the outbreak of schizophrenia had a temporal relationship with 'surgery of ovaries, pregnancy, delivery and puerperium'. Finally, Manfred Bleuler noted that late-onset schizophrenia (with onset after age 40 years) was much more frequent in women than in men, a finding he attributed to the 'loss of ovarian function' starting at around that age [4].

Basic Research Findings

Important findings from basic research revealed estrogen receptors in the limbic system of the brain, and the observation that the effects of estrogens in rodents are, in some respects, similar to those of neuroleptics. Furthermore, it was shown that estrogens can modulate the sensitivity and number of dopamine receptors. It was therefore hypothesized that estrogens exert their antipsychotic effects in a manner similar to that of traditional neuroleptics, at least partly via blockade of dopaminergic transmission [4].

In addition, it has been documented that estrogens, and especially 17β-estradiol (the natural estrogen that is most active in the brain), produce many other neuroprotective and psychoprotective effects. For example, estrogens appear to improve cerebral blood flow and glucose metabolism, promote neuronal sprouting and myelination, enhance synaptic density and plasticity, facilitate neuronal connectivity, act as antioxidants, and inhibit neuronal cell death. Estrogens also exert profound effects on brain differentiation during development, particularly during late gestation and during the early postnatal period, and are important in normal maintenance of brain function during aging [2].

The mechanism of action of estrogens depends not only on the classical genomic pathway, but also involves nongenomic, rapid interactions, which explains the differing latency of effects. Estrogens clearly modulate the dopaminergic and other neurotransmitter systems that are believed to be relevant to schizophrenia, such as the serotonergic and glutamergic system, but also the noradrenergic and cholinergic system [2]. Recently, it has even been suggested that 17β-estradiol in the brain might rather be regarded as a neurotransmitter itself than as a hormone [5].

There are at least two subtypes of estrogen receptors, namely estrogen receptor-α and estrogen receptor-β, which are transcribed from two distinct genes. Autopsy studies showed that estrogen receptor-α messenger RNA is expressed in discrete areas of the human brain such as amygdala, hypothalamus, cerebral cortex and hypocampus; these areas are associated with neuroendocrine function, as well as emotion, memory and cognition [2].

Epidemiological and Clinical Findings

Epidemiological studies of sex differences in schizophrenic disorders suggest that high estradiol production in young fertile women may contribute to the later age of onset in women compared to men, and to a better course of the disease especially in young women. Various epidemiological studies show that among females the disease on average begins 4–5 years later than in men (age 20–24 in men, 25–29 in women) [3], interestingly, women also exhibit an additional peak after age 45. Therefore, it has been postulated that estrogens raise the vulnerability threshold for the outbreak of the disease [4]. According to this hypothesis, women are, to some degree, protected against schizophrenia between puberty and the menopause by their relatively high gonadal estrogen production during this period of time. Women would lose the protection of estrogens with the onset of estrogen fluctuations/decline, which could account for their second peak of illness onset after age 45. Clinically, psychotic symptomatology has been shown to increase pre- or perimenstrually, i.e. in the low estrogen phase of the cycle [1, 2]. We examined 32 acutely admitted women with schizophrenia with history of regular menstrual cycles, and observed an increase in admissions during the perimenstrual low estrogen phase of the cycle. Furthermore, during the admission of these patients, a significant association emerged between estradiol levels and psychiatric symptomatology: symptoms appeared to improve when estradiol levels rose, and vice versa [6].

Seeman [7] noted that women with schizophrenia in the fertile age group of 20–40 years need lower doses of neuroleptics than do men of comparable age of older women, even when body weight is controlled. Gattaz et al. [8] in a further study found evidence of a differential therapeutic response depending on the phase of the menstrual cycle.

During pregnancy when estrogen levels are about 200-fold higher than normal, chronic psychoses seem to improve, but there is a 20-fold excess of psychosis after delivery, when estrogen levels suddenly drop to normal [1, 2]. Psychoses associated with other forms of estrogen withdrawal such as after abortion, removal of a hydatiform mole, cessation of oral contraceptives, clomifene and tamoxifen administration (both estrogen receptor antagonists) and gonadorelin agonist administration (blocking pituitary stimulation of endogenous estrogen secretion) have also been described [9].

Menopause and Schizophrenia

In a study of a large representative population of 392 first-admitted patients [10], we were able to show that the incidence of schizophrenia in the age group 40–60 years was about double in women, compared with men. First admission for schizophrenia after age 40 occurred in only 10% of all men with schizophrenia, but in about 21% of all women with this diagnosis. The yearly incidence rate in women over age 40 was 8.9 per 100,000, whereas it was only 4.2 per 100,000 in men [10] (fig. 1).

Interesting findings have been reported with respect to symptomatology and disease course of these late-onset women: *Men with onset over age 40* show significantly milder symptoms and spend less time in hospital than do early-onset patients, whereas late-onset women suffer from a disease that is almost as severe as that of patients who fall ill early in life [10]. An explanation for this could again be the estrogen effects: if onset of illness in women with a relative high vulnerability is delayed by estrogens, this high vulnerability is 'unmasked' by the loss of this estrogen protection around the time of the menopause. These women therefore are not only more frequently represented in the late-onset group but also have more severe symptoms and a worse course of illness. In addition, the depletion of dopamine receptors with age seems to be more precipitous in men than in women.

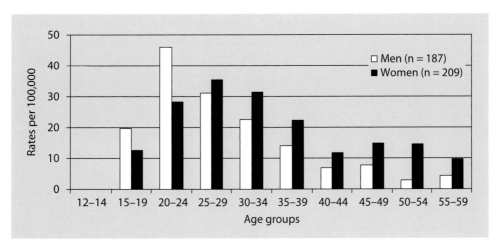

Fig. 1. Sex-specific age-distribution of first admissions because of schizophrenia and paranoid psychosis. From Häfner et al. [3].

Well in line with this are the results of long-term schizophrenia studies which have shown that the course of schizophrenia in women tends to deteriorate during the peri- and postmenopause [1, 2].

Intervention Studies with Estrogens

Intervention studies with estrogens have been conducted in women with schizophrenia of all age groups. As early as the 1940s, Bleuler [11] reported the first unsystematic trials using a combination of ovarian and pituitary hormones. Mall [12], a German psychiatrist in charge of a large hospital, examined 167 women suffering from schizophrenia with respect to estrogen excretion in a 24-hour urine sample, basal temperature and vaginal cytology. Based on his findings, he divided the psychoses into two groups: hypofollicular and hyperfollicular. In the former group, he replaced estrogens and found that 'hypofollicular psychosis can be healed relatively easily by this substitution therapy'.

Also, several contemporary investigators have now reported promising results using estrogen as a therapeutic agent. Ahokas et al. [13] demonstrated positive effects of estrogen substitution in two women with postpartum psychosis, and Sichel et al. [14] noted a prophylactic effect concerning this disorder. In a Cochrane review in 2005, Chua et al. [15] could only find five randomized double-blind intervention studies with a satisfying methodology, with most studies showing weak or nonsignificant effects. However, most of these studies employed conjugated estrogens rather than 17β-estradiol – the latter show to have pivotal activity in the brain. Furthermore, in order to prevent endometrial hyperplasia, the estrogens were usually combined with progestogens which can counteract the positive effects of estradiol in the brain.

Kulkarni et al. [16] found that schizophrenic women receiving estradiol as an adjunct to neuroleptic treatment showed more rapid improvement in psychotic symptoms than women receiving neuroleptics alone. In a recent randomized, double-blind study, the same group [17] showed that adjunctive transdermal estradiol significantly reduced positive and general psychopathological symptoms.

Most studies were conducted in young, premenopausal women. Only Good et al. [18] examined *post*menopausal patients. He administered estradiol and progesterone to 14 women with schizophrenia, schizophreniform or schizoaffective disorder and found a significant improvement of negative symptoms within six months. There are also some case reports regarding positive results of HRT in postmenopausal women with schizophrenia. Bergemann et al. [19] reported a case of a woman with first onset of schizophrenia in the perimenopause. She experienced severe first-rank symptoms over several months, but refused antipsychotic treatment. As she was symptomatic and believed to be in the perimenopause, therapy with transdermal estradiol in combination with norethisterone acetate was initiated and led to an impressive remission of the psychotic symptoms.

Lindamer et al. [20] reported on a postmenopausal woman whose psychotic symptoms improved on estradiol as an adjunct to her antipsychotic therapy. In 2001, Lindamer et al. [21] studied a community sample of postmenopausal women with schizophrenia. Twenty-four women received hormone replacement therapy (HRT), 28 women had never received such therapy. Interestingly, the users of HRT needed a relatively lower average dose of antipsychotic medication and suffered from less severe negative symptoms.

Premature Menopause in Schizophrenia

Several studies suggested disturbances in the gonadal function and hypoestrogenism in younger women with schizophrenic psychoses, similar to a 'premature menopause' [1]. Menstrual irregularities and reduced estradiol, progesterone and gonadotropin (FSH, LH) blood levels throughout the menstrual cycle, as well as anovulation and reduced fertility are also reported.

In our own study of 32 acutely admitted schizophrenic women, there was a greater variation in cycle length and significantly lower estradiol and progesterone blood levels throughout their menstrual cycle compared with 29 controls. Fifty-six percent presumably suffered from anovulation, which is a much higher proportion than in the control patients where anovulation was suspected in only 19% [22].

These findings are probably a consequence of neuroleptic-induced hyperprolactinemia which is known to suppress gonadal function [23]. As hypoestrogenism was also observed before the introduction of neuroleptics, it is possible that also 'stress' associated with psychosis could induce hyperprolactinemia and the respective gonadal suppression.

Estrogens and Bipolar Disorder

Little is known about the impact of female reproductive hormones on the course of bipolar disorder. Freeman et al. [24] assessed 50 women with DSM-IV bipolar disorder with a structured clinical interview regarding the impact of reproductive events on the course of the illness. They found an increased risk of mood symptoms at times of reproductive events. 2/3 of the women with children experienced a postpartum mood episode (mainly depressive episode). 22 of the women were currently either peri- or postmenopausal. Twelve of these women reported worsening of mood, namely an increase in depressive symptoms, increased irritability, hypomania or mania and more frequent cycling. Women who were not using hormone replacement therapy (HRT) were significantly more likely to report worsening of symptoms during perimenopause/menopause than those who were using HRT.

Estrogens' Influence on 'Accompanying' Symptoms of Psychosis

Physiological estrogens as well as HRT might have further positive effects in the therapy of psychosis. Thus, they might have stress-protective properties and thereby buffer against relapses. Furthermore they seem to have positive effects on cognition which is important, since minor cognitive deficits are often one of the main obstacles for rehabilitation in the post-acute phase of the disease. Again, cognitive properties of estrogens appear to be more associated with 17ß-estradiol rather than CEE (conjugated equine estrogens) [25, 26].

Hormone Replacement Therapy?

Trials should be initiated on therapy with estrogens for women with schizophrenia *during and after the perimenopause* as an augmentation strategy to neuroleptic medication. Possibly, the dose of neuroleptics could then be reduced and the corresponding side effects minimized. Estrogen therapy could also attenuate perimenopausal complaints such as hot flushes, night sweats with sleep disturbances and general irritability (table 1), symptoms that could lead to general deterioration of the mental state and potentially provoke a psychotic episode. Nonetheless, it has been reported that women with schizophrenia are less likely to ever use HRT as compared to women without psychiatric diagnosis [27]. Further research on the benefits of HRT for schizophrenic patients is therefore overdue.

Some of the positive effects of estrogens have been questioned in the context of perimenopausal estrogen replacement by studies such as the WHI, Women's Health Initiative Study [29], the WHI-M, Women's Health Initiative Memory Study [25] or the HERS, Heart and Estrogen/Progestin Replacement Study [30]. However, the

Table 1. Some important effects of estrogen replacement [28, 31, 32]

Positive	Negative
Perimenopausal complaints ↓ Physical: hot flushes, genital discomfort, aging of collagen (skin, joints, intervertebral discs) Mental: depression, irritability, emotional lability ↓	Endometrial carcinoma ↑ if unopposed estrogens are administered (→ in women without hysterectomy always combine with progestogens!)
Risk of osteoporosis ↓	Risk of breast cancer ↑? (→ not in patients with a familiar or own risk and usually not longer than 7 years!)
Delay of cognitive decline/Alzheimer?	Risk of thrombosis and cerebral insult ↑? (→ no prescription for patients at risk!)
Cardiovascular protection? (if started right after menopause)	Cardiovascular risks (coronary heart disease/ artherosclerosis)↑? (→ start only within the first 10 years after menopause and not in patients with cardiovascular disease!)

WHI study has been criticized by many experts and by the International Menopause Society [31] mainly due to some methodological limitations, e.g. mean age of 63 years and high prevalence of cardiovascular risk factors at study entry. The WHI re-analyses [32] have shown that the cardiovascular complications may be reduced by an early start of replacement therapy. Thus, there appears to be a window of opportunity for the potential cardiovascular benefits with HRT when replacement therapy is started early after the menopause [28].

Low and ultra-low doses of estrogens have been recently suggested for HRT [31] with transdermal application showing less side effects – with doses of 17β-estradiol varying from 14 to 25 μg. Whether low and ultra-low doses would have beneficial effects on mental well-being remains unclear.

Alternatives to Hormone Replacement Therapy

Compounds with more specific and potent estrogenic activity in the brain as opposed to other tissues are needed as an alternative to HRT. This would not only minimize side-effects of hormonal therapy, but may also allow new therapeutic strategies in men. Possible candidates are the selective estrogen receptor modulators (SERMs), whose agonist or antagonist properties depend on the target tissue. The effects of the existing SERMs (e.g. tibolone, raloxifen) on the brain, however, remain poorly studied.

Management of Premature Menopause

With growing evidence of altered gonadal function and premature menopause in schizophrenic females, the investigation of these patients should include questions regarding menstrual irregularities, amenorrhea, loss of libido, anorgasmia, infertility and galactorrhea; if estrogen deficiency is suspected, prolactin levels should be monitored. Hyperprolactinemia can theoretically be caused by the disease itself and the accompanying stress, but also by neuroleptic treatment, and can lead to secondary suppression of physiological estrogen production. Thus, many women treated with neuroleptics could suffer from a partially iatrogenic 'early menopause', with all the accompanied consequences, i.e. osteoporosis, enhanced cardiovascular risk and cognitive disturbances. In the case of neuroleptic-induced hyperprolactinemia with secondary estrogen deficiency, medication could be switched to a different agent with little or no associated hyperprolactinemia (e.g. quetiapine, aripiprazol, clozapine or olanzapine). As an alternative, estrogens could be added as an adjunct therapy to standard neuroleptic medication.

Management of Hormone-Drug Interactions

Estrogens may increase the efficacy of chlorpromazine [33], phenothiazines [34] and other antipsychotics [7]. With declining estrogen levels around the menopause, some women might benefit from dose adjustments of antipsychotics.

Other Medical and Psychosocial Aspects of Menopause in Patients with Psychoses

Medical Aspects

After the menopause, women are generally at an increased risk of developing a variety of medical disorders. Women with schizophrenia are even at an excess risk for many conditions, due to physical inactivity, poor diet, excessive smoking. Long-term neuroleptic treatment may also contribute to heightened morbidity, i.e. higher risk for metabolic syndrome, osteopenia or even osteoporosis.

Tardive dyskinesia seems to be more common and more severe in elderly women than men and seems to increase with age [35]. It has been suggested that estrogen withdrawal may contribute to this observation. Furthermore, thyroid function may be altered after menopause and influence mental well-being. Other frequent co-occurring medical illnesses in schizophrenia include diabetes, respiratory ailments and cardiovascular problems.

Unfortunately, schizophrenia patients are at great risk for greater medical neglect. Lindamer et al. [27] found that middle-aged and older women with schizophrenia were less likely to have had pelvic examination and PAP smears or mammograms compared to women with no known diagnosis. Older schizophrenic women should therefore be carefully monitored regarding their physical health with routine physical check-ups including blood pressure, weight and laboratory tests (glucose, lipids, etc.), EEG, mammography and PAP smears.

Psychosocial Aspects

Women during menopausal transition are also often confronted with many psychosocial stressors such as changes in family roles and manifold losses. In many cases, women with diagnosis of schizophrenia usually have already a very small social network and quite often report loneliness and a lack of social support.

Treatment recommendations for women in this age group therefore should include psychosocial support, skills training, supported employment, social welfare, etc. Psychotherapy should not only pay special attention to the ongoing stressors and losses, but also to their subjective experience of the menopause including their physical symptoms, their fears and beliefs regarding the experienced changes, their femininity and sexuality.

Conclusions

The menopause transition endures an enhanced risk of first onset of schizophrenic psychoses. Postmenopause is associated with quite severe symptoms in psychotic women whereas the severity of symptoms tends to diminish in aging men. This observation should have many implications for the appropriate treatment strategy, which should consider not only the potential benefits of estrogen replacement but also the use of psychosocial interventions.

Promising studies suggest that the neuroprotective properties of estrogen could justify its use as an adjunctive strategy to traditional drug therapies in schizophrenia.

Consideration of the menopausal status should be part of standard clinical care for mentally ill women. The use of estrogens, however, should always be decided on the basis of an individual risk-benefit assessment [31] in close co-operation between psychiatrists and gynecologists.

References

1 Riecher-Rössler A: Estrogens and Schizophrenia; in Bergemann N, Riecher-Rössler A (eds): Estrogen Effects in Psychiatric Disorders. Wien, Springer, 2005, pp 31–52.
2 Riecher-Rössler A: Oestrogens and schizophrenia. Curr Opin Psychiatry 2003;187–192.
3 Häfner H, Riecher A, Maurer K, Fatkenheuer B, Löffler W, van der Heiden W, Munk-Jörgensen P, Strömgren E: Geschlechtsunterschiede bei schizophrenen Erkrankungen. Fortschr Neurol Psychiatr 1991;59:343–360.

4 Riecher-Rössler A, Häfner H: Schizophrenia and oestrogens: is there an association? Eur Arch Psychiatry Clin Neurosci 1993;242:323–328.

5 Balthazart J, Ball GF: Is brain estradiol a hormone or a neurotransmitter? Trends Neurosci 2006;29: 241–249.

6 Riecher-Rössler A, Häfner H, Stumbaum M, Maurer K, Schmidt R: Can estradiol modulate schizophrenic symptomatology? Schizophr Bull 1994;20:203–214.

7 Seeman MV: Interaction of sex, age and neuroleptic dose. Compreh Psychiatry 1983;24:125–128.

8 Gattaz WF, Vogel P, Riecher-Rössler A, Soddu G: Influence of the menstrual cycle phase on the therapeutic response in schizophrenia. Biol Psychiatry 1994;36:137–139.

9 Mahe V, Dumaine A: Oestrogen withdrawal associated psychoses. Acta Psychiatr Scand 2001;104:323–331.

10 Riecher-Rössler A, Löffler W, Munk-Jörgensen P: What do we really know about late-onset schizophrenia? Eur Arch Psychiatry Clin Neurosci 1997; 247:195–208.

11 Bleuler M: Die spätschizophrenen Krankheitsbilder. Neurology 1943;15:259–290.

12 Mall G: Diagnostik und Therapie ovarieller Psychosen. Z Ges Neurol Psychiatr 1960;155:250.

13 Ahokas A, Aito M, Turtiainen S: Association between oestradiol and puerperal psychosis. Acta Psychiatr Scand 2000;101:167–169.

14 Sichel DA, Cohen LS, Robertson LM, Ruttenberg A, Rosenbaum JF: Prophylactic estrogen in recurrent postpartum affective disorder. Biol Psychiatry 1995;38:814–818.

15 Chua WL, de Izquierdo SA, Kulkarni J, Mortimer A: Estrogen for schizophrenia. Cochrane Database Systematic Rev 2005;4:CD004719.

16 Kulkarni J, Riedel A, de Castella AR, Fitzgerald PB, Rolfe TJ, Taffe J, Burger H: Estrogen: a potential treatment for schizophrenia. Schizophr Res 2001;48:137–144.

17 Kulkarni J, de CA, Fitzgerald PB, Gurvich CT, Bailey M, Bartholomeusz C, Burger H: Estrogen in severe mental illness: a potential new treatment approach. Arch Gen Psychiatry 2008;65:955–960.

18 Good KP, Kopala LC, Martzke JS, Fluker M, Seeman MV, Parish B, Shapiro H, Whitehorne L. Hormone replacement therapy in postmenopausal women with schizophrenia: preliminary findings. Schizophr Res 1999;12:131.

19 Bergemann N, Abu-Tair F, Strowitzki T: Estrogen in the treatment of late-onset schizophrenia. J Clin Psychopharmacol 2007;27:717–720.

20 Lindamer LA, Lohr JB, Harris MJ, Jeste DV: Gender, estrogen, and schizophrenia. Psychopharmacol Bull 1997;33:221–228.

21 Lindamer LA, Buse DC, Lohr JB, Jeste DV: Hormone replacement therapy in postmenopausal women with schizophrenia: positive effect on negative symptoms? Biol Psychiatry 2001;49:47–51.

22 Riecher-Rössler A, Häfner H, Dütsch-Strobel A, Stumbaum M: Gonadal function and its influence on psychopathology: a comparison of schizophrenic and non-schizophrenic female inpatients. Arch Women's Mental Health 1998;1:15–26.

23 Maguire GA: Prolactin elevation with antipsychotic medications: mechanisms of action and clinical consequences. J Clin Psychiatry 2002;63(suppl):56–62.

24 Freeman MP, Wosnitzer Smith K, Freeman SA, McElroy SL, Kmetz GF, Wright R, Keck PE: The impact of reproductive events on the course of bipolar disorder in women. J Clin Psychiatry 2002; 63: 284–287.

25 Craig MC, Maki PM, Murphy DG: The Women's Health Initiative Memory Study: findings and implications for treatment. Lancet Neurol 2005;iv:190–194.

26 Sherwin BB: Estrogen and memory in women: how can we reconcile the findings? Horm Behav 2005; 47:371–375.

27 Lindamer LA, Buse DC, Auslander A, Unutzer J, Bartels SJ, Jeste DV: A comparison of gynecological variables and services use in older women with and without schizophrenia. Psychiatr Serv 2003;54:902–904.

28 Riecher-Rössler A, de Geyter C: The forthcoming role of treatment with oestrogens in mental health. Swiss Med Wkly 2007;137:565–572.

29 Rossouw JE, Anderson GL, Prentice RL, LaCroix AZ, Kooperberg C, Stefanick ML, Jackson RD, Beresford SA, Howard BV, Johnson KC, Kotchen JM, Ockene J: Risks and benefits of estrogen plus progestin in healthy postmenopausal women: principal results From the Women's Health Initiative randomized controlled trial. JAMA 2002;288:321–333.

30 Hlatky MA, Boothroyd D, Vittinghoff E, Sharp P, Whooley MA: Quality-of-life and depressive symptoms in postmenopausal women after receiving hormone therapy: results from the Heart and Estrogen/Progestin Replacement Study (HERS) trial. JAMA 2002;287:591–597.

31 Birkhäuser MH, Panay N, Archer DF, Barlow D, Burger H, Gambacciani M, Goldstein S, Pinkerton JA, Sturdee DW: Updated practical recommendations for hormone replacement therapy in the peri- and postmenopause. Climacteric 2008;11:108–123.

32 Rossouw JE, Prentice RL, Manson JE, Wu L, Barad D, Barnabei VM, Ko M, LaCroix AZ, Margolis KL, Stefanick ML: Postmenopausal hormone therapy and risk of cardiovascular disease by age and years since menopause. JAMA 2007;297:1465–1477.

33 Martin E: Drug Interactions Index 1978/1979. Philadelphia, Lippincott, 1978.

34 Hanslen P: Drug Interactions, ed 3. Philadelphia, Lea & Febiger, 1976.

35 Seeman MV, Fitzgerald P: Women and schizophrenia: clinical aspects; in Castle D, McGrath J, Kulkarni J (eds): Women and Schizophrenia. Cambridge, Cambridge University Press, 2000, pp 35–50.

Prof. Dr. med. Anita Riecher
Psychiatric Outpatient Department, University Hospital Basel
Petersgraben 4
CH–4031 Basel (Switzerland)
Tel. +41 61 265 51 14, Fax +41 61 265 45 99, E-Mail ariecher@uhbs.ch

Soares CN, Warren M (eds): The Menopausal Transition. Interface between Gynecology and Psychiatry.
Key Issues in Mental Health. Basel, Karger, 2009, vol 175, pp 127–144

Hormone Therapies and Menopause: Where Do We Stand in the Post-WHI Era?

Michelle P. Warren[a] · Kanani E. Titchen[a] · Meir Steiner[b,c]

[a]Center for Menopause, Hormonal Disorders and Women's Health, Columbia University Medical Center, New York, N.Y., USA; [b]McMaster University, Hamilton, Ont., and [c]Department of Psychiatry and Institute of Medical Sciences, University of Toronto, The Hospital for Sick Children, Toronto, Ont., Canada

Abstract

The WHI study, its premature termination, and controversy over its findings have motivated patients and physicians alike to seek lower-dose therapies for menopausal symptoms. Substantial data indicate that low-dose ET/EPT is effective in treating osteoporosis, hot flushes, vulvaginal dryness and itching, and sleeping difficulties. Furthermore, low-dose therapies are associated with a decrease in breast tenderness compared to standard dose therapies. Some risks associated with standard-dose HT diminish with low-dose treatments. Risk of stroke and venous thromboembolism, for example, fall to placebo levels with low-dose therapies. The nebulous effects on breast cancer and colorectal cancer rates, as well as on risk of CHD, point to the need for further study of low-dose therapies. In light of suggestions that timing of HT may play a role in a therapy's efficacy and safety, more study of perimenopausal and younger postmenopausal patients is warranted. Such therapy should be started as close to the onset of menopause as possible. In addition, recent data suggest that hormone therapy should currently be limited to the lowest dose possible for the duration of time needed to alleviate menopausal symptoms and should be in accordance with the patient's medical history and risk status.

Background

Although life expectancy for North-American women has almost doubled in the past century, age of onset of menopause has remained unchanged [1]. As a result, far more women are living longer with menopausal symptoms, including – but by no means limited to – the following: hot flashes; vulvovaginal atrophy, itching, irritation, and drying; painful intercourse; onset or worsening of osteoporosis; headaches and myalgia; vasomotor and sleep disturbances; increased coronary heart disease (CHD) risk; depression, melancholia, nervousness, and/or irritability [2–8].

The clinical use of estrogens to treat menopausal symptoms was first described nearly 80 years ago [9]. In the early 1940s, oral estrogen formulations for postmenopausal hormone therapy became available and since that time doses of estrogen in hormone therapy have been decreasing [10]. Until the mid-1970s, daily doses of conjugated equine estrogens (CEE) as high as 1.25 or 2.5 mg were commonly used [11], thereafter transitioning to 0.625 mg/day as the standard dose for estrogen therapy (ET) [12]. The accompanying progestin dose of 2.5 mg was similarly adopted as standard in combined estrogen progestin therapy (EPT) [13].

Women's Health Initiative

Early Termination

In 2002, the initial results reported from the Women's Health Initiative (WHI) indicated that 5 years of standard-dose EPT decreased a woman's risk of fracture but increased her risk of coronary heart disease, stroke, venous thromboembolism (VTE), and breast cancer [14]. Due primarily to concerns about an increasing hazard ratio (HR) for incident breast cancer, the WHI-EPT trial was stopped prematurely. It was reported that the 'overall health risks exceeded benefits from use of combined estrogen plus progestin ... among healthy postmenopausal US women' [14].

Furthermore, the estrogen-only study (WHI-CEE) was stopped a year prematurely, with the WHI citing an increased risk of stroke in the absence of any cardiovascular benefit [15]. Although a slight reduction in breast cancer was observed with estrogen-alone therapy, it was not found to be significant. A reduction in hip fractures was also observed in women aged 60 and older. Nonetheless, citing the 'burden of incident disease events', the WHI investigators shut down the WHI-CEE arm of the study [15].

Despite the very small risks, the reports led many women to discontinue hormone therapy – some temporarily and some permanently. The ramifications of stopping and re-starting hormone treatment are currently the subject of much study, and it will likely take years to uncover the effects on women's health of the WHI study and its early termination.

Design

An ambitious study involving over 161,000 female subjects (16,608 in the estrogen plus progestin component alone), the WHI focused attention on women's health and hormone therapy as a possible agent to prevent heart disease as no other study had done before it [14]. Details of the study design and data analysis, however, have undergone much scrutiny and criticism since the study's premature end. For example, the study population averaged more than 63 years of age: this threw into doubt the ability to generalize the results to all postmenopausal women, and particularly women entering the menopause [16, 17].

Additionally, the initiation and administration of standard EPT doses to post-menopausal women in their mid-60s to mid-70s did not reflect common clinical practice. These were women whose final menstrual periods were decades ago and whose bodies had long ceased to produce 17β-estradiol, the primary ovarian estrogen product in menstruating women. The results from the ET trial of the WHI [18] and more recent age-stratified analyses from the EPT trial [19–21] provide good evidence that the risk-benefit profile of standard-dose ET and EPT is significantly more favorable in younger postmenopausal women, i.e. those who initiate ET/EPT within a few years following their final menstrual period, than that observed in the overall WHI study population [22–24].

In addition to age range differences, confounding factors such as smoking, hypertension, and obesity may have influenced study outcomes. The average study participant was overweight (average BMI = 28) with one third qualifying as obese (BMI ≥30). One third of the participants were hypertensive, an eighth were on medications for high cholesterol, and fully half of all participants had a history of smoking [14]. How, then, are we to extrapolate data gathered from an unhealthy older menopausal population to a younger healthy one?

WHI Data Are Contradicted

Several other large observational studies gathered evidence contradicting results presented by the WHI. For instance, in the Nurses' Health Study (NHS) involving 121,700 female nurses, women with no prior history of CHD who used hormone therapy (HT) experienced a 30–50% reduction in CHD compared to HT never users [20]. Estrogen, then, would appear to have beneficial effects on the cardiovascular system. What accounts for the reversal in CHD findings? The WHI-EPT arm reported an increased risk of CHD, while the WHI-CEE arm reported no change in CHD. Is estrogen beneficial, harmful or simply not a factor where CHD is concerned?

In each of these studies, patient population characteristics must be considered: In general, WHI patients were older and more overweight, were more likely to smoke, and were less likely to use aspirin than those in the NHS [14, 20]. It is possible then that WHI patients had already begun to develop atherosclerosis, a condition that may diminish the protective cardiovascular effect of estrogen [25].

In fact, the biological effects exerted by estrogen have been found to differ for atherosclerotic vessels versus healthy ones in animal (including primate) studies [26–30]. Therefore, according to the 'timing hypothesis', hormone therapy may be effective in preventing atherosclerosis in humans only when it is initiated prior to or during menopause, before advanced atherosclerosis has developed. A sub-study of the WHI data (known as the WHI-CACS) supports the timing hypothesis, stating that for a

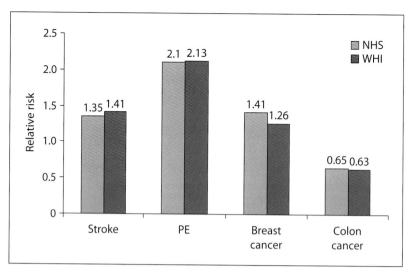

Fig. 1. Relative risks of the WHI vs. the NHS [14, 20, 25].

younger subset of women 'the mean coronary-artery calcium score after trial completion was lower among women receiving estrogen (83.1) than among those receiving placebo (123.1)' [31]. This follow-up analysis of 1,064 women from the WHI cohort found that female 50- to 59-year-olds adherent to the estrogen regimen experienced a 61% reduction in coronary calcification compared to those on placebo [24, 31]. Again, population age and time since menopause play a crucial role in disease outcome.

Regarding effect of HT on mortality, the most marked reduction in specific causes of death in the NHS was in death due to coronary heart disease (RR 0.47). This, too, supports the idea that estrogen has positive effects on cardiovascular health in younger, healthy postmenopausal women. Thus, estrogen alone – if started at menopause – may protect the heart [31].

WHI Data Are Supported

In other areas, data in support of the WHI results were found. As an example, NHS results for stroke, pulmonary embolism (PE), colon cancer and breast cancer were consistent with WHI (fig. 1).

Additionally, the Framingham Study, involving 2,873 postmenopausal women, reported that risks of both colon cancer and hip fracture were attenuated by unopposed estrogen, once again in agreement with the WHI. Relative risks were 0.34 for hip fracture in women who had taken estrogens within the past 2 years and 0.65 in women who had ever taken estrogens [32]. The WHI study yielded similarly reduced fracture hazard ratios (0.61 for hip fracture and 0.70 for overall fracture in women in the CEE group) [15, 33].

Just one type of hormone therapy – the standard EPT dose of 0.625 CEE and 2.5 mg medroxyprogesterone acetate (MPA) – was used in the WHI study; from this, sweeping conclusions were drawn regarding the safety and efficacy of all hormone therapies and all doses. As pointed out by Ettinger nearly a decade ago, the assumption that there exists a single dose of estrogen (or progestin, for that matter) that will relieve all menopausal symptoms and prevent bone loss is probably incorrect. Rather, a continuum of positive changes on symptoms and bone density is to be expected, with no threshold minimal dose, as was once believed [12]. Recent data related to bone mineral density (BMD) and plasma estradiol concentrations supports this position. Where plasma estradiol concentrations of at least 180 pmol/l (49 pg/ml) were long believed to be necessary to prevent vertebral bone loss, a recent study by Genant et al. [34] determined that mean plasma levels of just 90 pmol/l (24.5 pg/ml) were associated with significant increases in spinal BMD.

The WHI declared the objective of its study 'to assess the major health benefits and risks of the most commonly used combined hormone preparation in the United States' [18]. The study, however, provided little information about menopausal symptom relief or quality of life (QOL) in symptomatic women, arguably two important aspects of 'health benefits' for menopausal women. Instead, the study prioritizes one health ailment or disease over another; for instance, breast cancer risk over osteoporosis and fracture-risk. As Utian [35] writes, 'Any clinician who has spent time with patients suffering with various chronic diseases realizes that one disease is not equivalent to another. In this day and age, for example, it is far easier – medically and emotionally – for the majority of women to be treated for early-stage breast cancer than to be immobilized by severe backache following osteoporotic vertebral crush fractures'.

Quality of life, then, must be taken into account when considering the risk/benefit ratio of hormone therapy. Using the Greene Climacteric Scale, Barentsen et al. [36] found that anxiety, somatic symptoms (i.e. headaches, dizziness, myalgia), vasomotor episodes, and sexual interest worsened significantly in postmenopausal women when compared to premenopausal women. Although these conditions are generally not life-threatening, each plays a significant role in women's quality of life. Furthermore, some symptoms persist for years – even decades.

Kronenberg [37], for example, showed that women sometimes suffer hot flushes, a non-life threatening but highly disruptive condition, for more than 20 years. A survey of 501 postmenopausal women ranging in ages from 29 to 82 years, revealed that flushing could last from just a few months to as many as 44 years after menopause. While approximately 60% of these women suffered hot flushes for fewer than 7 years, 15% experienced them for more than 15 years. One of the primary complaints of women with hot flushes is a disruption in sleep. Women may awaken drenched in sweat several times during the night, resulting in fatigue and irritability the following day [37, 38]. In fact, the correlation between disrupted sleep and menopause-related mood changes has been well documented by several researchers [39, 40] but not by all [41]. Thus, the effects of hot flushes may indirectly extend beyond the physical symptoms and prove disruptive to a woman's psychological well-being. Even if menopause per se may not be a strong predictor of specific sleep-disorder symptoms as measured by polysomnography, women in midlife are less satisfied with their sleep [42].

In short, the WHI study serves as an incomplete but significant exploration into the effects of hormone therapy on disease in the older, postmenopausal female population. Another study of its size and scope is unlikely to take place again in the near future. For this reason alone, it is disappointing that the trial was stopped short of its proposed 8.5-year duration, thereby diminishing the precision of long-term treatment effect estimates. The study fails to address short-term effects of hormone therapy on menopausal symptoms, and results from the WHI study cannot be generalized to lower dosages of EPT, to other routes of administration (i.e. transdermal), nor to other ET/EPT formulations. The Writing Group for the WHI Investigators has stated that 'no noteworthy interactions with age … were found for the effect of estrogen plus progestin on CHD, stroke, or VTE,' but no allowance for time-since-onset-of-menopause is made [18]. Further study is needed to ascertain the risks and benefits of HT as a function of time-since-menopause.

Hormones: Risks and Benefits

The WHI study did draw attention to some of the risks of standard dose hormone therapy, especially when newly administered many years after a woman's final menstruation. Risk of cardiovascular heart disease (CHD), for instance, does increase with EPT, patient's age, and the number of years since menopause – when all of these factors are considered together [43]. WHI-EPT findings concerning a small increase in breast cancer, too, were largely supported by the Million Women's Study (MWS), an observational study which reported a correlation between current EPT use and increased risk of breast cancer [44]. On the other hand, the MWS reported a small increase in breast cancer with estrogen alone, while the WHI reported none after 7.1 years of unopposed CEE [15, 44].

When discussing the risks of HT, however, clinicians must translate relative risks into absolute risks. As an example, the WHI study estimated a total hazard ratio (or relative risk, RR) of 1.26 for HRT versus placebo at 5.2 years. This RR translates to eight additional breast cancer occurrences per 10,000 women per year. When all the monitored outcomes are combined (heart attack, stroke, breast cancer, venous thromboembolism (VTE), colorectal cancer, and hip fracture,) women on HRT might expect 19 more events per year *per 10,000 women* than women on placebo [14]. A more recent meta-analysis parses by age group the number of events prevented and

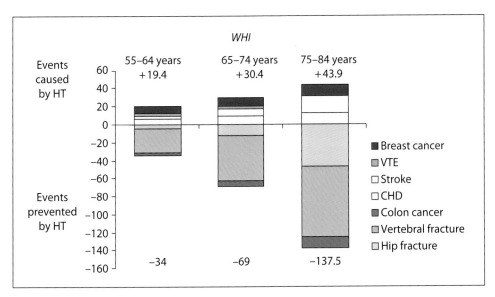

Fig. 2. HT use in 10,000 women: benefits and serious harm per year by age [14, 45].

caused by hormone therapy, contrasting the risk-to-benefit ratios derived from meta-analysis to those reported by the WHI [45]. This analysis favors by a considerable margin benefits versus risk (fig. 2).

In discussing risks of HT, it is also imperative that clinicians distinguish between risks associated with estrogen alone (ET) and those associated with estrogen plus pro-gestin (EPT). For instance, the WHI study estimated an HR of 0.77 for invasive breast cancers among the women using ET [46]. Contrast this to an HR of 1.26 for invasive breast cancers among women in the EPT group [18].

Even in the light of these small risks, HT remains underutilized in the United States, with fewer than 30% of postmenopausal women using it. For those women who do initiate therapy, compliance tends to be poor, due largely to breakthrough bleeding and fears of breast cancer and weight gain [47, 48]. In contrast, most women achieve amenorrhea from continuous-combined regimens within 1 year of starting hormone therapy. Furthermore, fears of risks and side effects tend to be exaggerated. For example, 61% of respondents in a telephone survey of 1,000 US women identified all cancers as the greatest health problem confronting women (34% identifying breast cancer, specifically). In fact, a far lower 19% of women aged 65 and older actually die of any form of cancer. Paradoxically, just 7% of women in this same survey identified cardiovascular disease as women's greatest health problem; in reality, heart disease is the leading cause of death among US women 65 and older, accounting for 34% of total deaths. These statistics highlight menopausal patients' misperceptions of their greatest health problems and underscore the need for patient education and physician continuing education so that women and their doctors can make more educated deci-sions about hormone therapy.

Lastly, the benefits from using ET/EPT might well exceed risks, depending on the patient's age, lifestyle, and medical history. Considerable symptomatic relief is afforded by ET/EPT, as will be discussed later. Estrogen therapy, especially when started during the menopausal transition or soon after menopause, is associated with reduced rates of fracture and colon cancer, and these benefits may be strengthened when accompanied by necessary changes to patient lifestyle and medical care [14, 20, 49]. According to a recent meta-analysis, estrogen therapy may not be able to attenuate all of the effects of aging which continue to contribute to osteoporosis and fractures [45]. Ethnicity is also likely to be a factor with some groups, such as Caucasians, demonstrating greater risk [50, 51].

Cessation of Hormone Therapy

For Those Women Who Stopped Their Hormone Therapy Regimens in Response to the WHI, What Are the Consequences?

In summary, both the risks and the benefits of hormone therapy are reversible upon discontinuation. Cessation of EPT after several years of use is associated with a reversal in the trends of increased breast cancer, cardiovascular events, deep vein thrombosis and pulmonary embolism. In a follow-up study to the WHI, each of these risks was attenuated 2.4 years after women discontinued hormone use. Similarly, beneficial effects of EPT abated: the reduced colorectal cancer risk associated with CEE plus MPA disappeared, and risks of fractures were nearly equal between EPT and placebo groups within 2.4 years after stopping therapy (HR 0.91 for the EPT group) [52].

Interestingly, breast cancer risk diminished over time after EPT use, while *overall* risk of total malignancies *increased* upon cessation of EPT from 1.03 HR during treatment to 1.24 HR 2.4 years after stopping treatment. This surprising increase in malignancy risk after stopping treatment was attributed to an attenuation of estrogen's protection against colon cancer. The reduced colorectal cancer risk observed in the EPT group increased from 0.62 HR during treatment to 1.08 post-EPT; thus, the protective effects of EPT against colorectal cancer vanished 2.4 years after discontinuing hormone use [52]. Conversely, cancers *other* than breast, endometrial, ovarian, and colorectal cancers were responsible for a large number of absolute mortalities, and most cancer-related deaths were due to lung cancers. Endometrial cancer rates in the EPT group were lower than in the placebo group, but this difference did not reach statistical significance. Thus, as the protective effects on colon cancer were lost, the decrease in breast cancer risk was replaced by an increase in a combination of other malignancies, in particular lung cancer. The physiologic reasons for this are unclear and may be more related to lifestyle than to EPT use.

Low-Dose Hormone Therapy

Even before the discontinuation of the WHI hormone therapy trials, strong interest in the safety and efficacy of lower doses of ET and EPT was evident [14, 18]. Use of the lowest effective dose of any medication remains an important tenet of clinical practice and is a worthwhile goal in the treatment of the postmenopausal patient [53]. Consistent with this goal, current guidelines around the world unanimously recommend the use of the lowest effective dose of ET/EPT [54–57]. What, then, constitutes low-dose hormone therapy?

Low-dose ET is currently defined as oral conjugated equine estrogen (CEE) 0.45 mg/day or less, oral estradiol 0.5 mg/day or less, or transdermal estradiol 0.025 mg/day or less, or an equivalent; but tablet formulations containing as little as 0.3 mg of CEE are available. Transdermal E_2 patches that deliver as little as 0.014 mg per day are also available, although their FDA-allowed use is limited to prevention of osteoporosis since further study is needed to ascertain any vulvovaginal benefit [58].

Endometrial thickening, produced by standard doses of estrogen, correlates to irregular vaginal bleeding, which for many women is a leading reason for poor compliance with therapy [34, 59–62]. Lower doses of estrogen are associated with higher rates of amenorrhea and a lower incidence of uterine bleeding compared with standard-dose therapy [62–68]. Use of lower estrogen doses has the added benefit of allowing use of lower progestin doses to protect the endometrium of women with an intact uterus [34, 59, 60, 69]. As of this writing, a low-dose combination patch is not yet commercially available, but several other combination EPT products are. Low-dose oral CEE (0.45 or 0.3 mg/day) is commonly combined with low-dose (1.5 mg/day) MPA; similarly, 0.5 mg/day oral E_2 is available in combination with low-dose norethisterone acetate (NETA, 0.1 mg/day). In addition, multiple combinations of low dose hormones are now in use with two-pill therapy.

Applications of Low-Dose Hormone Therapies

The decision to opt for one hormone therapy regimen over another will depend upon the chief complaint of the patient, pre-existing health conditions, and approved uses or proven efficacies of the therapy. The latter will be reviewed here.

Vasomotor symptoms are shown to be alleviated by low ET/EPT therapies [70]. A review of studies reporting vasomotor symptom relief comparing low-dose estrogens to placebo found that hot flashes experienced by patients in active treatment groups were reduced by 65% [71]. Of note is that low-dose EPT regimens have been reported to relieve vasomotor symptoms as effectively as standard doses. Alternatively, unopposed low-dose CEE formulations are effective but perhaps less so, showing a slight dose-related effect [72]. Data from the Women's Health, Osteoporosis, Progestin, Estrogen (HOPE) study, which evaluated the additive effect of progestin (1.5 mg/day

MPA) to low-dose oral CEE, support this discrepancy between ET and EPT in relieving vasomotor symptoms.

Vulvovaginal atrophy, as measured by the vaginal maturation index (VMI), is effectively reduced by low-dose CEE with or without MPA in younger postmenopausal women (mean age 52.4 years) [72]. Although correlation of the VMI to symptoms associated with vaginal atrophy is debated, other studies support this claim of reduced vulvovaginal atrophy in response to low-dose therapies. For instance, reductions in vaginal dryness scores were achieved with 0.5 mg/day 17β-estradiol with either 0.1 mg or 0.25 mg NETA, again in relatively young postmenopausal women [73]. Preliminary evidence suggests that low-dose transdermal estradiol (14 μg/day) may alleviate vulvovaginal atrophy in women with an intact uterus (mean age = 67 years), but transdermal E_2 at this dose is not currently indicated for relief of vaginal symptoms [61]. Further study is needed.

Alternatively, local therapies (i.e. vaginal creams) are effective and can be added to low-dose therapy with little to no systemic absorption [74–76].

Bone mineral density (BMD) measured at the lumbar spine in postmenopausal women (mean age = 51.1 to 51.9 years) has been shown to increase with just a 14-μg/day transdermal E_2 patch (the Menostar patch, FDA approved for this purpose alone), with both standard-dose (0.625 mg/day) and low-dose (0.3 mg/day) oral CEE, and with low-dose oral CEE (0.3 and 0.45 mg/day) administered alone or with MPA (1.5 and 2.5 mg/day). Positive effects of 0.3 mg CEE with 2.5 mg MPA on spinal BMD were also found in postmenopausal women >65 years of age with low bone mass [77]. In fact, in a healthy population of women >65 years (n = 83), low-dose oral 17β-estradiol (0.25 mg/day) increased BMD of the hip, spine, and total body, and reduced bone turnover compared to placebo (n = 84). No differences in BMD were evident between non-hysterectomized women (61%) receiving EPT and those who received ET alone [78]. Overall, studies indicate that low doses of ET/EPT effectively prevent bone loss [67]. Regardless of the ET/EPT regimen chosen, supplementation with 1,200–1,500 mg of oral calcium and 400–800 IU vitamin D per day is recommended for postmenopausal women aged 51 and over [55].

The incidence of *colorectal cancer* began to decline after 3 years of treatment with standard dose EPT, with significant differences between the EPT and placebo groups becoming more pronounced with time. These results were consistent with observational studies, as reported by Grodstein et al. [20] in the late 1990s. The effects of lower dose therapies remain to be seen.

Other potential benefits of lower-dose ET/EPT regimens have been well documented. Compared to placebo, a combination of low-dose oral E_2 (0.5 mg/day) with NETA (0.1 or 0.25 mg/day) correlated to significantly less difficulty sleeping, as measured by the Greene Climacteric Scale [73]. In women ≥65 years who were on low-dose oral E_2 (0.25 mg/day) for 3 years, no effects have been found on skeletal muscle mass, physical functioning, and body fat when compared with placebo [79]. In a 2-year study using 14 μg/day transdermal E_2, no effect on cognitive function

– positive or negative – was suggested by results on cognitive test scores when compared with placebo [80]. Breast tenderness is a side effect of ET/EPT that appears to be dose-related, and lower doses of estrogen are associated with a lower incidence of breast tenderness [63, 66–68].

On the other hand, estrogen therapies have been associated with increased breast tissue density, which might put women at greater risk for breast cancer [81–84]. Some investigators have proposed that dense breast tissue diminishes mammographic sensitivity, making mammograms more difficult to read and resulting in more missed cancers [85–87]. To date, however, the increased risk has been associated only with baseline breast density. Furthermore, women on HT tend to get mammograms more frequently, thereby increasing the likelihood of early detection.

A number of methods are currently being developed and refined in an effort to estimate breast cancer risk based on breast density [88–90]. On the other hand, breast density alone cannot provide complete breast cancer risk assessment: family history, ethnicity, risk-associated behaviors (i.e. smoking), and disease associated with hereditary breast cancer can all play a role. Risk estimates, therefore, should 'be combined with the potential benefits and harms of tests and treatments (along with a woman's preference for those tests and treatments) to make the best clinical decisions for individual patients' [88].

Safety

Important when contemplating any medication is an understanding of the drug's safety profile. Hormone therapies, whether natural or synthetic, are no different, and extensive data regarding safety exist for standard and lower dose HTs.

The risk of *venous thromboembolism* (VTE) increases with standard dose ET/EPT [14, 18]. Preliminary evidence suggests that lower dose ET/EPT may reduce this risk [91, 92]. It has been suggested that route of estrogen administration could also affect VTE risk [93]. The Estrogen and Thromboembolism Risk (ESTHER) study group found a 4-fold increase in risk of VTE for oral estrogen users compared to nonusers and transdermal estrogen users (mean age = 61.5 years) [93]. It is important to note, however, that doses of transdermal and oral estrogen were not equivalent, with roughly 85% of transdermal users receiving ≤0.050 mg/day (equivalent to approximately 1.0 mg/day oral) and oral users receiving an average of 1.5 mg/day [93]. Significantly larger studies are warranted, however, to clarify the differences between standard and low-dose hormone therapy and route of administration where VTE is concerned.

Stroke risk appears to increase with use of standard-dose estrogen use, according to a number of observational studies as well as the ET/EPT arms of the WHI study [20, 94, 95]. The Nurses' Health Study goes one step further, relating the risk of stroke to the daily dose of estrogen: Women using standard doses of CEE or higher had a significantly increased risk of stroke compared to women not using estrogen, whereas women using low-dose CEE (0.3 mg/day) showed no increase in risk [20]. Additional research is needed in this area to determine both the impact of dosing and the impact of route of administration (RA) on stroke risk.

Breast cancer risk was found to increase slightly in women using standard-dose EPT (containing 2.5 mg/day medroxyprogesterone acetate) in the WHI study. This increase was not seen in hysterectomized women using unopposed estrogen [14, 18]. The Women's Health Study, in contrast to the Women's Health Initiative, revealed that breast cancer risk increased with estrogen dose but not progestin dose and cited a 0.87 RR for breast cancer with low-dose therapy [96]. Thus, an increase in breast cancer risk is observed with progesterone but not with progestin therapy. The role of estrogen dosing on breast cancer risk remains elusive: two other large studies found no effect [97, 98]. In addition, some studies have demonstrated that women using HT are less likely to develop metastases and are likely to live longer than women who have not used HT [99]. This is in line with data gathered separately by Fournier et al. [100] and Bardou et al. [101] indicating that women using HT developed more ER+ tumors, which are associated with better overall health and survival compared to ER– tumors,.

An analysis of the Nurses' Health Study by Chen et al. [102] sought to parse out the association between long-term ET use and breast cancer risk in postmenopausal women. The analysis was limited to postmenopausal women who had undergone hysterectomy; thus, these women did not require progestogen therapy in conjunction with ET. Investigators noted a linear increase in invasive breast cancer risk with increased duration of ET. However, the relative risk (RR) did not demonstrate statistical significance until use of ET exceeded 20 years, and women using ET for 10 years or less were not at any greater risk for breast cancer (RR 0.96) [102].

As Fournier notes, it is important to remember that neither breast cancer nor hormone therapy is a single entity. Just as tumors remain distinct in regard to their hormone receptors and histologies, so do hormone therapies vary in their dosages, routes of administration, and chemical structures [100]. Currently, little evidence addresses the effect of lower ET/EPT doses on breast cancer risk.

Cardiovascular heart disease (CHD) risk, as mentioned previously, decreases with standard-dose ET/EPT use for those women who initiate therapy at the time of menopause and for those women who have no history of or predisposition toward CHD [19, 31, 103] Little is known about the effect of low-dose and transdermal HT regimens on CHD.

Younger Women: Are the Risks the Same?

The WHI study brought to the world's attention the myriad health challenges and risks faced by older postmenopausal women. Do these risks and benefits translate to younger women?

As discussed earlier, the risks to older postmenopausal women (>60 years) do not necessarily apply to postmenopausal women in their 40s and 50s or to women who are perimenopausal. Studies have shown that the number of years since menopause plays a crucial role in determining risks and benefits of hormone therapies. In short, the benefit-to-risk ratio increases in younger peri- and postmenopausal women. Nonetheless, postmenopausal HT should be prescribed at the lowest effective dose for the shortest amount of time consistent with treatment goals for women aware of potential risks and benefits, and provided there is clinical supervision [104]. Furthermore, according to the North American Menopause Society (NAMS,) data from the WHI study 'should not be extrapolated to symptomatic postmenopausal women younger than 50 years of age who initiate HT at that time, as these women were not studied in those trials' [104].

Benefits also tend to outweigh risks in premenopausal women with premature ovarian failure (POF). POF, unlike menopause, can be characterized by a highly irregular menstrual cycle rather than a complete stopping of menses. If untreated, the result is menopausal symptoms – namely, hot flashes and night sweats, lethargy, irritability, painful intercourse, and vaginal atrophy and drying. POF is also associated with premature osteoporosis and increased cardiovascular morbidity and mortality. Hormone therapy has proven an effective treatment for the vasomotor symptoms, vaginal atrophy, and bone loss in patients with POF [105–107].

Alternative Therapies

What Options Are Available for Women who Should Not or Will Not Take Hormone Therapy?
Custom-Compounded HTs, based on a woman's specific needs and hormone panel/profile, have proven no safer than standard and mass-produced regimens. Granted, there is a dearth of evidence due to the lack of controlled clinical trials of safety and efficacy. Such studies are unlikely to be attempted due to their high costs and lack of patent protection [108]. Claims that these hormones are safer are unfounded.

Nonprescription remedies, such as dietary isoflavones, black cohosh, dong quai, and vitamin E, are typically tested in the short-term only and demonstrate little efficacy over placebo. Nonetheless, these are generally safe alternatives, with no evidence of harm to the consumer [109–111].

Lifestyle changes including a reduction in alcohol and caffeine intake, avoidance of spicy foods, cessation of smoking, and manipulation of ambient temperature have shown to be slightly effective. Again, these are safe alternatives and may confer added benefits, such as the reduction in risk of cardiovascular disease that accompanies a nonsmoking lifestyle [109–111].

Selective serotonin uptake inhibitors (SSRIs) and *gabapentin* have demonstrated some abatement of vasomotor symptoms in preliminary studies [112,113]. A

Canadian study has demonstrated that the decrease in the number of HRT prescriptions was associated with a statistically significant increase in prescriptions of serotonergic antidepressants, suggesting that SSRIs are being prescribed for symptoms previously controlled with the use of HRT [114].

Clonidine, an antihypertensive α-adrenergic receptor agonist commonly prescribed for insomnia, anxiety, and substance abuse withdrawal, has also demonstrated efficacy in this area [109–111]. *Bisphosphonates, selective estrogen receptor agonists* (SERMs), and *calcitonin* are common treatments for the osteoporotic symptoms that accompany endogenous estrogen loss, whether due to post-oopherectomy or naturally occurring menopause. As stated previously, a regimen of calcium with vitamin D should accompany these treatments.

Phytoestrogens, including isoflavones, lignans, and coumestans, are nonsteroidal plant-based chemicals that exhibit estrogen-like activity.

Megestrol acetate, in the class of progestogens (synthetic progesterones), is used to treat breast cancer. Progestogens and their uses, however, are now suspect in light of WHI findings; consideration, therefore, must be given to concurrent therapies that may further impede estrogen-dependent processes in the body (i.e. bone remodeling) [115, 116].

References

1 US Department of Health and Human Services: Healthy People 2010. Federal Interagency Forum on Aging-Related Statistics. Washington, 2000.

2 Guthrie JR, Dennerstein L, Taffe JR, Lehert P, Burger HG: The menopausal transition: a 9-year prospective population-based study. The Melbourne Women's Midlife Health Project. Climacteric 2004;7: 375–389.

3 Cohen LS, Soares CN, Vitonis AF, Otto MW, Harlow BL: Risk for new onset of depression during the menopausal transition: the Harvard study of moods and cycles. Arch Gen Psychiatry 2006;63:385–390.

4 Leiblum SR, Koochaki PE, Rodenberg CA, Barton IP, Rosen RC: Hypoactive sexual desire disorder in postmenopausal women: US results from the Women's International Study of Health and Sexuality (WISHeS). Menopause 2006;13:46–56.

5 Versi E, Harvey MA, Cardozo L, Brincat M, Studd JW: Urogenital prolapse and atrophy at menopause: a prevalence study. Int Urogynecol J Pelvic Floor Dysfunct 2001;12:107–110.

6 Brincat M, Kabalan S, Studd JW, Moniz CF, de TJ, Montgomery J: A study of the decrease of skin collagen content, skin thickness, and bone mass in the postmenopausal woman. Obstet Gynecol 1987;70: 840–845.

7 Sowers MR, Jannausch M, McConnell D et al: Hormone predictors of bone mineral density changes during the menopausal transition. J Clin Endocrinol Metab 2006;91:1261–1267.

8 Sowers M, Derby C, Jannausch ML, Torrens JI, Pasternak R: Insulin resistance, hemostatic factors, and hormone interactions in pre- and perimenopausal women: SWAN. J Clin Endocrinol Metab 2003;88:4904–4910.

9 Severinghaus EL, Evans JS: Clinical observations on the use of an ovarian hormone: anmoitin. Am J Med Sci 1929;178:638–645.

10 Warren MP: Historical perspectives in postmenopausal hormone therapy: defining the right dose and duration. Mayo Clin Proc 2007;82:219–226.

11 Lobo RA, Whitehead MI: Is low-dose hormone replacement therapy for postmenopausal women efficacious and desirable? Climacteric 2001;4:110–119.

12 Ettinger B: Personal perspective on low-dosage estrogen therapy for postmenopausal women. Menopause 1999;6:273–276.

13 Gambrell RD, Jr: Strategies to reduce the incidence of endometrial cancer in postmenopausal women. Am J Obstet Gynecol 1997;177:1196–1204.

14 Writing Group for the Women's Health Initiative Investigators: Risks and benefits of estrogen plus progestin in healthy postmenopausal women: principal results from the Women's Health Initiative randomized controlled trial. JAMA 2002;288:321–333.

15 Anderson GL, Limacher M, Assaf AR, et al: Effects of conjugated equine estrogen in postmenopausal women with hysterectomy: the Women's Health Initiative randomized controlled trial. JAMA 2004; 291:1701–1712.

16 Bhavnani BR, Strickler RC: Menopausal hormone therapy. Journal of Obstetrics and Gynaecology Canada 2005;27:137–162.

17 Lobo RA, Belisle S, Creasman WT, et al: Should symptomatic menopausal women be offered hormone therapy? MedGenMed 2006;8:1.

18 Women's Health Initiative Steering Committee: Effects of conjugated equine estrogen in postmenopausal women having undergone hysterectomy: The Women's Health Initiative Randomized, Controlled Trials. Obstet Gynecol Surv 2004;59:599–600.

19 Rossouw JE, Prentice RL, Manson JE, et al : Postmenopausal hormone therapy and risk of cardiovascular disease by age and years since menopause. JAMA 2007;297:1465–1477.

20 Grodstein F, Manson JE, Colditz GA, Willett WC, Speizer FE, Stampfer MJ: A prospective, observational study of postmenopausal hormone therapy and primary prevention of cardiovascular disease. Ann Intern Med 2000;133:933–941.

21 Chlebowski RT, Hendrix SL, Langer RD et al: Influence of estrogen plus progestin on breast cancer and mammography in healthy postmenopausal women: the Women's Health Initiative randomized trial. JAMA 2003;289:3243–3253.

22 Burger HG: WHI risks: any relevance to menopause management? Maturitas 2007;57:6–10.

23 Salpeter S: Hormone therapy for younger postmenopausal women: how can we make sense out of the evidence? Climacteric 2005;8:307–310.

24 Mendelsohn ME, Karas RH: HRT and the young at heart. N Engl J Med 2007;356:2639–2641.

25 Colditz GA, Hankinson SE, Hunter DJ, et al: The use of estrogens and progestins and the risk of breast cancer in postmenopausal women. N Engl J Med 1995;332:1589–1593.

26 Haarbo J, Christiansen C: The impact of female sex hormones on secondary prevention of atherosclerosis in ovariectomized cholesterol-fed rabbits. Atherosclerosis 1996;123:139–144.

27 Clarkson TB, Appt SE: Controversies about HRT–lessons from monkey models. Maturitas 2005;51:64–74.

28 Hanke H, Kamenz J, Hanke S, et al: Effect of 17-beta estradiol on pre-existing atherosclerotic lesions: role of the endothelium. Atherosclerosis 1999;147:123–132.

29 Mendelsohn ME: Protective effects of estrogen on the cardiovascular system. Am J Cardiol 2002;89: 12E–7E.

30 Mendelsohn ME, Karas RH: Molecular and cellular basis of cardiovascular gender differences. Science 2005;308:1583–1587.

31 Manson JE, Allison MA, Rossouw JE, et al: Estrogen therapy and coronary-artery calcification. N Engl J Med 2007;356:2591–2602.

32 Kiel DP, Felson DT, Anderson JJ, Wilson PW, Moskowitz MA: Hip fracture and the use of estrogens in postmenopausal women. The Framingham Study. N Engl J Med 1987;317:1169–1174.

33 Jackson RD, Wactawski-Wende J, LaCroix AZ, et al: Effects of conjugated equine estrogen on risk of fractures and BMD in postmenopausal women with hysterectomy: results from the women's health initiative randomized trial. J Bone Miner Res 2006; 21:817–828.

34 Genant HK, Lucas J, Weiss S, et al: Low-dose esterified estrogen therapy: effects on bone, plasma estradiol concentrations, endometrium, and lipid levels. Arch Intern Med 1997;157:2609–2615.

35 Utian WH: NIH and WHI: time for a mea culpa and steps beyond. Menopause 2007;14:1056–1059.

36 Barentsen R, van de Weijer PH, van GS, Foekema H: Climacteric symptoms in a representative Dutch population sample as measured with the Greene Climacteric Scale. Maturitas 2001;38:123–128.

37 Kronenberg F: Hot flashes: epidemiology and physiology. Ann NY Acad Sci 1990;592:52–86.

38 Ohayon MM: Severe hot flashes are associated with chronic insomnia. Arch Intern Med 2006;166:1262–1268.

39 Shaver JL, Zenk SN: Sleep disturbance in menopause. J Womens Health Gend Based Med 2000; 9:109–118.

40 Baker A, Simpson S, Dawson D: Sleep disruption and mood changes associated with menopause. J Psychosom Res 1997;43:359–369.

41 Manson JE, Hsia J, Johnson KC et al: Estrogen plus progestin and the risk of coronary heart disease. N Engl J Med 2003;349:523–534.

42 Kalleinen N, Polo-Kantola P, Himanen SL, Alhola P, Joutsen A, Urrila AS, Polo O: Sleep and the menopause: do postmenopausal women experience worse sleep than premenopausal women? Menopause Int 2008;3:97–104.

43 Young T, Rabago D, Zgierska A, AustinD, Laurel F: Objective and subjective sleep quality in premenopausal, perimenopausal, and postmenopausal women in the Wisconsin Sleep Cohort Study. Sleep 2003;6:667–672.

44 Beral V: Breast cancer and hormone-replacement therapy in the Million Women Study. Lancet 2003; 362:419–427.

45 Nelson HD, Humphrey LL, Nygren P, Teutsch SM, Allan JD: Postmenopausal hormone replacement therapy: scientific review. JAMA 2002;288:872–881.

46 Women's Health Initiative Steering Committee: Effects of conjugated equine estrogen in postmenopausal women with hysterectomy: the Women's Health Initiative randomized controlled trial. JAMA 2004;291:1701–1712.

47 Ravnikar VA: Compliance with hormone replacement therapy: are women receiving the full impact of hormone replacement therapy preventive health benefits? Womens Health Issues 1992;2:75–80.

48 Goldman GA, Kaplan B, Leiserowitz DM, Pardo Y, Amster R, Fisch B: Compliance with hormone replacement therapy in postmenopausal women: a comparative study. Clin Exp Obstet Gynecol 1998;25:18–19.

49 Nelson HD, Rizzo J, Harris E, et al: Osteoporosis and fractures in postmenopausal women using estrogen. Arch Intern Med 2002;162:2278–2284.

50 Dawson-Hughes B, Tosteson AN, Melton LJ III, et al: Implications of absolute fracture risk assessment for osteoporosis practice guidelines in the USA. Osteoporos Int 2008;19:449–458.

51 Robbins J, Aragaki AK, Kooperberg C, et al: Factors associated with 5-year risk of hip fracture in postmenopausal women. JAMA 2007;298:2389–2398.

52 Heiss G, Wallace R, Anderson GL, et al: Health risks and benefits 3 years after stopping randomized treatment with estrogen and progestin. JAMA 2008;299:1036–1045.

53 Archer DF: Lower doses of oral estrogen and progestogens as treatment for postmenopausal women. Semin Reprod Med 2005;23:188–195.

54 Skouby SO, Al-Azzawi F, Barlow D, et al: Climacteric medicine: European Menopause and Andropause Society (EMAS) 2004/2005 position statements on peri- and postmenopausal hormone replacement therapy. Maturitas 2005;51:8–14.

55 American College of Obstetricians and Gynecologists: ACOG practice bulletin. Clinical management guidelines for obstetrician-gynecologists. Obstet Gynecol 2004;103:203–216.

56 North American Menopause Society: Estrogen and progestogen use in peri- and postmenopausal women: March 2007 position statement of The North American Menopause Society. Menopause 2007;14:168–182.

57 Maia H Jr, Albernaz MA, Baracat EC, et al: Latin American position on the current status of hormone therapy during the menopausal transition and thereafter. Maturitas 2006;55:5–13.

58 Berlex: Menostar® (Berlex) 2004.

59 Ettinger B: Rationale for use of lower estrogen doses for postmenopausal hormone therapy. Maturitas 2007;57:81–84.

60 Pickar JH, Yeh I-T, Wheeler JE, Cunnane MF, Speroff L: Endometrial effects of lower doses of conjugated equine estrogens and medroxyprogesterone acetate. Fertil Steril 2001;76:25–31.

61 Johnson SR, Ettinger B, Macer JL, Ensrud KE, Quan J, Grady D: Uterine and vaginal effects of unopposed ultralow-dose transdermal estradiol. Obstet Gynecol 2005;105:779–787.

62 Archer DF, Dorin M, Lewis V, Schneider DL, Pickar JH: Effects of lower doses of conjugated equine estrogens and medroxyprogesterone acetate on endometrial bleeding. Fertil Steril 2001;75:1080–1087.

63 Prestwood KM, Kenny AM, Unson C, Kulldorff M: The effect of low dose micronized 17b-estradiol on bone turnover, sex hormone levels, and side effects in older women: a randomized, double blind, placebo-controlled study. J Clin Endocrinol Metab 2000;85:4462–4469.

64 Symons J, Kempfert N, Speroff L: Vaginal bleeding in postmenopausal women taking low-dose norethindrone acetate and ethinyl estradiol combinations. Obstet Gynecol 2000;96:366–372.

65 Utian WH, Burry KA, Archer DF et al: Efficacy and safety of low, standard, and high dosages of an estradiol transdermal system (Esclim) compared with placebo on vasomotor symptoms in highly symptomatic menopausal patients. Am J Obstet Gynecol 1999;181:71–79.

66 Notelovitz M, Lenihan JP Jr, McDermott M, Kerber IJ, Nanavati N, Arce J-C: Initial 17b-estradiol dose for treating vasomotor symptoms. Obstet Gynecol 2000;95:726–731.

67 Speroff L, Rowan J, Symons J, Genant H, Wilborn W: The comparative effect on bone density, endometrium, and lipids of continuous hormones as replacement therapy (CHART Study): a randomized controlled trial. JAMA 1996;276:1397–1403.

68 van de Weijer PH, Mattsson LA, Ylikorkala O: Benefits and risks of long-term low-dose oral continuous combined hormone therapy. Maturitas 2006;56:231–248.

69 Pickar JH, Yeh I-T, Wheeler JE, Cunnane MF, Speroff L: Endometrial effects of lower doses of conjugated equine estrogens and medroxyprogesterone acetate: two year substudy results. Fertil Steril 2003;80:1234–1240.

70 Maclennan AH, Broadbent JL, Lester S, Moore V: Oral oestrogen and combined oestrogen/progestogen therapy versus placebo for hot flushes. Cochrane Database Syst Rev 2004;4:CD002978.

71 Ettinger B: Vasomotor symptom relief versus unwanted effects: role of estrogen dosage. Am J Med 2005;118:1407–1408.

72 Utian WH, Shoupe D, Bachmann G, Pinkerton JV, Pickar JH: Relief of vasomotor symptoms and vaginal atrophy with lower doses of conjugated equine estrogens and medroxyprogesterone acetate. Fertil Steril 2001;75:1065–1079.

73 Panay N, Ylikorkala O, Archer DF, Gut R, Lang E: Ultra-low-dose estradiol and norethisterone acetate: effective menopausal symptom relief. Climacteric 2007;10:120–131.

74 Raymundo N, Yu-cheng B, Zi-yan H, et al: Treatment of atrophic vaginitis with topical conjugated equine estrogens in postmenopausal Asian women. Climacteric 2004;7:312–18.

75 Mandel FP, Geola FL, Meldrum DR, et al: Biological effects of various doses of vaginally administered conjugated equine estrogens in postmenopausal women. J Clin Endocrinol Metab 1983;57:133–139.

76 Notelovitz M, Funk S, Nanavati N, Mazzeo M: Estradiol absorption from vaginal tablets in postmenopausal women. Obstet Gynecol 2002;99:556–562.

77 Recker RR, Davies KM, Dowd RM, Heaney RP: The effect of low-dose continuous estrogen and progesterone therapy with calcium and vitamin D on bone in elderly women: a randomized, controlled trial. Ann Intern Med 1999;130:897–904.

78 Prestwood KM, Kenny AM, Kleppinger A, Kulldorff M: Ultra low-dose micronized 17b-estradiol and bone density and bone metabolism in older women: a randomized controlled trial. JAMA 2003;290:1042–1048.

79 Kenny AM, Kleppinger A, Wang Y, Prestwood KM: Effects of ultra-low-dose estrogen therapy on muscle and physical function in older women. JAGS 2005;53:1973–1977.

80 Yaffe K, Vittinghoff E, Ensrud KE, et al: Effects of ultra-low-dose transdermal estradiol on cognition and health-related quality of life. Arch Neurol 2006;63:945–950.

81 Saftlas AF, Wolfe JN, Hoover RN et al: Mammographic parenchymal patterns as indicators of breast cancer risk. Am J Epidemiol 1989;129:518–526.

82 Boyd NF, Byng JW, Jong RA, et al: Quantitative classification of mammographic densities and breast cancer risk: results from the Canadian National Breast Screening Study. J Natl Cancer Inst 1995;87:670–675.

83 Boyd NF, Lockwood GA, Byng JW, Tritchler DL, Yaffe MJ: Mammographic densities and breast cancer risk. Cancer Epidemiol Biomarkers Prev 1998;7:1133–1144.

84 Wolfe JN, Saftlas AF, Salane M: Mammographic parenchymal patterns and quantitative evaluation of mammographic densities: a case-control study. AJR Am J Roentgenol 1987;148:1087–1092.

85 Kerlikowske K, Grady D, Barclay J, Sickles EA, Ernster V: Effect of age, breast density, and family history on the sensitivity of first screening mammography. JAMA 1996;276:33–38.

86 van Gils CH, Otten JD, Verbeek AL, Hendriks JH: Mammographic breast density and risk of breast cancer: masking bias or causality? Eur J Epidemiol 1998;14:315–320.

87 van Gils CH, Otten JD, Verbeek AL, Hendriks JH, Holland R: Effect of mammographic breast density on breast cancer screening performance: a study in Nijmegen, The Netherlands. J Epidemiol Commun Health 1998;52:267–271.

88 Tice JA, Cummings SR, Smith-Bindman R, Ichikawa L, Barlow WE, Kerlikowske K: Using clinical factors and mammographic breast density to estimate breast cancer risk: development and validation of a new predictive model. Ann Intern Med 2008;148:337–347.

89 Barlow WE, White E, Ballard-Barbash R et al: Prospective breast cancer risk prediction model for women undergoing screening mammography. J Natl Cancer Inst 2006;98:1204–1214.

90 Chen J, Pee D, Ayyagari R et al: Projecting absolute invasive breast cancer risk in white women with a model that includes mammographic density. J Natl Cancer Inst 2006;98:1215–1226.

91 Jick H, Derby LE, Myers MW, Vasilakis C, Newton KM: Risk of hospital admission for idiopathic venous thromboembolism among users of postmenopausal oestrogens. Lancet 1996;348:981–983.

92 Lobo RA: Evaluation of cardiovascular event rates with hormone therapy in healthy, early postmenopausal women: results from 2 large clinical trials. Arch Intern Med 2004;164:482–484.

93 Canonico M, Oger E, Plu-Bureau, et al: Hormone therapy and venous thromboembolism among postmenopausal women: impact of the route of estrogen administration and progestogens: the ESTHER study. Circulation 2007;115:840–845.

94 Hendrix SL, Wassertheil-Smoller S, Johnson KC, et al: Effects of conjugated equine estrogen on stroke in the Women's Health Initiative. Circulation 2006;113:2425–2434.

95 Wassertheil-Smoller S, Hendrix S, Limacher M, et al: Effect of estrogen plus progestin on stroke in postmenopausal women: The Women's Health Initiative: a randomized trial. JAMA 2003;289:2673–2684.

96 Porch JV, Lee IM, Cook NR, Rexrode KM, Burin JE: Estrogen-progestin replacement therapy and breast cancer risk: the Women's Health Study (United States). CCC 2002;13:847–854.

97 Million Women Study Collaborators: Breast cancer and hormone-replacement therapy in the Million Women Study. Lancet 2003;362:419–427.

98 Collaborative Group on Hormonal Factors in Breast Cancer. Breast cancer and hormone replacement therapy: collaborative reanalysis of data from 51 epidemiological studies of 52 705 women with breast cancer and 108 411 women without breast cancer. Lancet 1997;350:1047–1059.

99 Colditz GA, Egan KM, Stampfer MJ. Hormone replacement therapy and risk of breast cancer: results from epidemiologic studies. Am J Obstet Gynecol 1993;168:1473–1480.

100 Fournier A, Fabre A, Mesrine S, Boutron-Ruault MC, Berrino F, Clavel-Chapelon F: Use of different postmenopausal hormone therapies and risk of histology- and hormone receptor-defined invasive breast cancer. J Clin Oncol 2008;26:1260–1268.

101 Bardou VJ, Arpino G, Elledge RM, Osborne CK, Clark GM: Progesterone receptor status significantly improves outcome prediction over estrogen receptor status alone for adjuvant endocrine therapy in two large breast cancer databases. J Clin Oncol 2003;21:1973–1979.

102 Chen WY, Manson JE, Hankinson SE et al : Unopposed estrogen therapy and the risk of invasive breast cancer. Arch Intern Med 2006;166:1027–1032.

103 Grodstein F, Manson JE, Stampfer MJ: Hormone therapy and coronary heart disease: the role of time since menopause and age at hormone initiation. J Womens Health 2006;15:35–44.

104 Seifert-Klauss V, Kingwell E, Hitchcock CL, Kalyan S, Prior JC: Estrogen and progestogen use in peri- and postmenopausal women: March 2007 position statement of The North American Menopause Society. Menopause 2008;15:203–204.

105 Nelson LM, Covington SN, Rebar RW: An update: spontaneous premature ovarian failure is not an early menopause. Fertil Steril 2005;83:1327–1332.

106 Executive Summary: Hormone therapy. Obstet Gynecol 2004;104(suppl):1S–4S.

107 Estrogen and progestogen use in peri- and postmenopausal women: September 2003 position statement of The North American Menopause Society. Menopause 2003;10:497–506.

108 Boothby LA, Doering PL, Kipersztok S: Bioidentical hormone therapy: a review. Menopause 2004;11:356–367.

109 Treatment of menopause-associated vasomotor symptoms: position statement of The North American Menopause Society. Menopause 2004;11:11–33.

110 Kronenberg F, Fugh-Berman A: Complementary and alternative medicine for menopausal symptoms: a review of randomized, controlled trials. Ann Intern Med 2002;137:805–813.

111 Huntley A, Ernst E: A systematic review of the safety of black cohosh. Menopause 2003;10:58–64.

112 Cheema D, Coomarasamy A, El-Toukhy T: Non-hormonal therapy of post-menopausal vasomotor symptoms: a structured evidence-based review. Arch Gynecol Obstet 2007;276:463–469.

113 Warren MP: Missed symptoms of menopause. Int J Clin Pract 2007;61:2041–2050.

114 McIntyre RS, Konarski JZ, Grigoriadis S, Fan NC, Mancini DA, Fulton KA, Stewart DE, Kennedy SH: Hormone replacement therapy and antidepressant prescription patterns: a reciprocal relationship. CMA J 2005;172:57–59.

115 Kuhl H: Pharmacology of estrogens and progestogens: influence of different routes of administration. Climacteric 2005;8 (suppl):3–63.

116 Sitruk-Ware R: New progestogens: a review of their effects in perimenopausal and postmenopausal women. Drugs Aging 2004;21:865–883.

Michelle P. Warren, MD
Center for Menopause, Hormonal Disorders and Women's Health, Columbia University Medical Center
622 W. 168th Street, PH 16–128
New York, NY 10032 (USA)
Tel. +1 212 305 8723, Fax +1 212 305 9945, E-Mail mpw1@columbia.edu

Author Index

Subject Index